How to Burn Body Fat Completely and Maintain a Slim Physique Permanently

Nekoterran

From the Author:

I want to thank you and congratulate you for purchasing the book *How to Burn Body Fat Completely and Maintain a Slim Physique Permanently.*

This book contains proven steps and strategies on how to lose the weight from head to toe and keep a fit physique forever.

In this program, you will learn unmatched wisdom in weight loss that doesn't exist anywhere else.

The weight loss community, like the bodybuilding community, has got losing weight incomplete and in many areas incorrect.

This is why you are searching for answers…and now you have finally come to the right place.

IF YOU FOLLOW THESE PRINCIPLES, YOU ARE GURANTEED TO BURN BODY FAT COMPLETELY AND MAINTAIN A SLIM PHYSIQUE PERMANENTLY.

Thanks again for purchasing this book. I hope you take the information in, and APPLY what you learn to your fitness routine and life.

CONTENTS:

If you enjoy this book do consider leaving a review…

www.nekoterran.com/advice

Read together with…

Basic Internal Detox

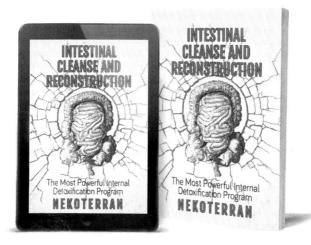

- ✓ Deep internal detoxification program.
- ✓ This is the ideal program to begin with.
- ✓ Complete this program first before attempting weight loss or bodybuilding basics
- ✓ Works in conjunction with every other program.

Introduction:

I am not a fitness instructor, nor do I have a coaching license.

The information in this program is not tailored to replace your current workout routine or diet. The weight loss has not been evaluated by the AFAA, Medical Fitness Association, American Sports and Fitness Association, IDEA Health & Fitness Association or any other fitness association.

All the information you will learn is based on direct experience and experimentation on myself, my bodybuilding peers, fitness enthusiasts and the average overweight individual who also achieved outstanding results.

Be warned:

IF YOU FOLLOW THESE PRINCIPLES, YOU ARE GURANTEED TO BURN BODY FAT COMPLETELY AND MAINTAIN A SLIM PHYSIQUE PERMANENTLY.

However, it is possible that the techniques outlined have some measure of risk, like everything in this world. You must use common sense and consult with your physician or fitness instructor if necessary prior to the workouts and dietary principles. You, the reader alone, is the only one responsible for the methods outlined in this program.

To illustrate a point:

From Earl Nightingale, *The Strangest Secret in the World:*

During the 1950s, a survey was made in the USA of one hundred working men aged 25.

The survey contained two questions:

1. Do you want to be rich?
2. Will you be rich?

Without a moment of hesitation, all one hundred men answered "Yes!" and "Yes!" Every single one of them were eager towards life. They had a positive attitude towards the world. There was a certain sparkle in their eyes, radiating assuredness of a bright and abundant future.

But do you know what happened?

By the time they reached the age of 65, one man became rich, four were financially independent, forty-five were still working and fifty were broke.

But why?

What happened to the dreams, hopes and ambitions?

The answer is because of goals.

What about the rest of the 95 working men?

Believe it or not, 19 out of 20 men do not know why they wake up every morning. They just exist, adapt and play along with their surroundings. The 95% who do not have goals, or any sense of direction, don't have a choice but to conform.

Except for the top few, the majority play the world's most undesirable yet common game known as "follow the follower."

The problem is that most follow the wrong group—the unsuccessful 95%—and suffer the same consequences.

Successful individuals started like everyone else: at the bottom. Successful people know they must stand out, think out of the box, and take control of their own lives.

Rich people didn't become rich out of luck, or talent or occult knowledge. Those who are at the top decided to earn more. They made it their business to earn more. And as a result, they became rich.

Decision (goal) + learn how + take constructive action = success

The harsh reality is that 19 out of 20 of these working men have seldom if ever done any constructive thinking on how they will earn more money, or in other words, increase their income.

If a person doesn't decide to cook tomato sauce spaghetti for dinner (goal), she will never look up the recipe (learn how to), or be able to prepare or cook (take constructive action) tomato sauce spaghetti.

Only 1 out 20 (top 5%) men have actually made it their business to earn more money. Just thinking about their goal will lead to zero. The rich took action towards their goal. They decided to become rich. They learned how to earn more money. They studied the recipes of "how" to become rich, and as a result, they made more money.

In your case:

Decide to burn body fat completely and maintain a slim physique permanently + learn how + act on what you learn = a slim physique

Since only 5% of people know what they desire (goal), all 5% can and will be winners. In this race, there aren't even enough contestants to contend against. Even the runner who comes in last can be a winner.

And the rest of the 95% will always remain where they are.

What does this illustration have to do with weight loss?

If you choose to belong to the top 5%, then the time has come to try a new approach—a completely different approach that will separate you from the rest and deliver results without harming the body in any way shape or form.

At your local gym, or any gym anywhere on this planet, out of one hundred clients, regardless of their age, who experience working out and years spent doing cardio, how many have the physique they desire?

One or two? Or none?

Just like the example above, chances are that only 5% or less acquire the physique of their choice.

Why?

Most have been programmed for years with weight loss advice from their peers (who don't have a clue how to burn body fat), fitness instructors (who learned how to build muscle, and burn body fat from previous trainers whose source of information come from fitness magazines that are over a decade old), or a weight loss website written by a random ghostwriter, and so on.

Most-searched topic in the world:

Two of the most-searched topics on the internet are "how to lose weight" and "how to lose body fat."

There are hundreds, if not thousands, of fitness and weight loss magazines, books, websites, nutritional guides, TV programs, fitness instructors, weight loss gurus, etc.

If there is so much information on weight loss, why is there so much controversy on the topic? Shouldn't everyone at the gym or on a diet obtain the results they are after?

But the results speak for themselves...

The answer is simple:

The weight loss community, just like the bodybuilding community, has the information incorrect or incomplete!

Think of this:

Muscle and Fitness magazine was first published in 1936 by Joe Weider. If you compare side by side a bodybuilding magazine from the 1970s, 1980s, 1990s, 2000, and 2010, it will become evident that the workout instructions, nutrition facts, and diets plans are completely contrasting.

Why is the information drastically changing?

Because the bodybuilding community cannot accurately pin down once and for all what builds muscle and burns fat.

4

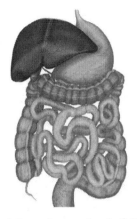

Think about what occurs inside the body to build muscle, accumulate fat or burn excess body fat.

Only a selective few have the physique they desire because the information available is incorrect or incomplete. Like most who follow the wrong crowd on autopilot without questioning or without a second thought, they will suffer the same consequences. Unfortunately, this is the plain and simple truth.

Most who carelessly follow gym instructors, trainers, overweight peers, and magazine ghost writers who do not have a clue why body fat accumulates in the first place will be led to a dead end.

You may be thinking:

Really? Are you sure?

To find out for yourself, conduct your own survey. Ask people inside and outside the gym, personal whoever else question #1.

1. **What happens INSIDE the body to accumulate excess fat?**

    After you evaluate the *ummm* and the silent stare you get, ask question #2.

2. **How is a slim physique maintained after excess body fat has been burnt off?**

    When the silence becomes too unnerving, move onto the next person.

    Ask 10 - 100 - 1,000 until you are 100% convinced that nobody has the physique, or ability to keep their physique in shape, because they don't know what builds muscle and causes body fat accumulation in the first place.

Out of the dozens of bodybuilders, ex-bodybuilders, fitness enthusiasts, therapists, certified nutritionists, kinesiologists, iridologists, registered dieticians, gymnasts, fitness nutrition certificate holders, doctors or anyone relevant to the subject matter I have asked/interviewed...not one person had an accurate understanding to the two simple questions.

To prove it, ask yourself these two questions.

<PAUSE>

If you answered, "I don't know," then that is why you struggle to lose weight.

Common weight loss programs popular today:

Paleo diet (caveman diet):

- Consuming large amounts of protein is acid-forming, and it is the worst source of fuel for the human body, and it interrupts the digestive process and clogs the stomach and intestines.

- Protein is the dirtiest source of fuel in the category of fats, carbohydrates, and proteins.

- Only a small amount of protein is necessary to repair muscle, and this amount is far less than you might realize.

- Humans aren't designed to eat meat—tigers and lions are.

- The paleo diet teaches to eat 4-6 small meals a day. This is by far the worst mistake, forcing the body to go into a chronic sugar-burning state.

Ketogenic diet:

- Carbohydrates are necessary for the body to function. Cutting out all carbohydrates, including the right carbohydrates, will lead to serious nutritional deficiencies.

- This diet is also too high in protein.
- Frequent small meals each day destroy the body.

Atkins diet:

- Cutting out all carbohydrates causes more damage than good.
- More protein than necessary does not burn body fat, but harms the body.
- Frequent small meals each day are harmful to the body.

Avoid carbs after 6 pm:

- Avoiding heavy meals during the body's cleansing cycle (evening and early morning) is correct. However, eating carbs after 6 pm alone is not the only cause of body fat accumulation.

Eat less and walk/exercise more:

- Eating less food is starvation.
- We all have to eat the right foods and cut out the wrong foods to lose weight and keep the weight of long-term.
- If you eat less than what the body requires, this approach will lead to disease and nutritional deficiencies. The whole point of eating is to live. To survive is the reason humans eat in the first place.
- If you observe those who follow the "eat less and walk/jog more" approach, they will always lack energy, eventually break down and binge eat or go back to bad habits, which leads to gaining all the weight back.

Burn more calories than consumed:

- This approach is the same idea as eating less and moving more.
- Do you know what calories are? How many calories are required?
- Definition of calorie: *the energy needed to raise the temperature of 1 kilogram of water through 1 °C, equal to one thousand small calories and often used to measure the energy value of foods.*
- ***What does this definition mean?***
- Has counting the number of calories worked?
- Energy is required for the body to function. Energy will never turn into body fat! Isn't this common sense?

Eat 4-6 small meals a day: (by FAR the most terrible mistake!)

- Eating 4-6 small meals a day will force the body into a chronic sugar-burning state, which leads to muscle mass deterioration, loss of energy and causes excess body fat accumulation.

None of the methods above address the causes and reasons why excess body fat accumulates in the first place. The diets/routines above work marginally or are totally ineffective because they are incorrect or incomplete.

Let me repeat, if you don't know what/why/how body fat accumulates or what happens inside the body to build muscle, you can never get rid of body fat or build muscle!

This is obvious. This is common sense.

What is in this program?

If you are unhappy with your body, KNOW that an unhealthy physique has a cause. All disease, excess fat accumulation, and unhealthy physique have causes.

Excess fat accumulation doesn't amass on its own. If you have attempted to burn body fat for months or years, and don't see the results you are after, there is a reason. If you know exactly what causes fat to accumulate in the first place and what prevents further fattening, and if you learn how to burn body fat, strengthen/tone muscle fibers, and maintain muscle mass from deterioration, you will then achieve the physique you have always dreamed of. This is common sense.

My story:

For over 10 years after high school, I read every fitness book and *Muscle & Fitness* magazine; I adopted instructions from pro and ex-bodybuilders, took courses from fitness coaches, and attempted every weight loss diet and fitness program; I jogged, cycled and did bodyweight workout. Everything and anything that I could find on building muscle mass and weight loss I did.

However, regardless of how many hours I spent at the gym, or whichever strict diet I followed, I still couldn't build muscle or burn fat. My body didn't change whatsoever!

After years of no results, I grew so unhappy, depressed and hopeless with my body that I wanted to give up all together. Then I made the decision to take an unconventional route, an unknown course that would separate me from the rest.

To make a long story short, I began to do some serious research. RE-search is just as it sounds; it means searching again. None of the information in this book I came up with on my own.

I chose to abandon the traditional bodybuilding routines, diets, protein powders, supplements, etc., and instead studied the mechanics of the human body. In other words, the internal functions of how the human body works. From whichever relevant source…anything and everything that makes sense…I have done. After following through everything the bodybuilding and fitness community had to

9

offer, at one point, I decided to end this pointless cycle all together.

For months, I collected whatever information was available and tested everything on myself. As a result, I put together 4 programs:

1) How to burn body fat completely and maintain a slim physique permanently.

2) How to build more muscle than ever before and maintain muscle mass permanently.

3) Intestinal cleanse and reconstruction—the most powerful detoxification program.

4) How to build a monstrous physique for the extreme hardcore bodybuilder.

In a few short weeks of applying the principles, my waist shrunk from 36 inches to 34 inches. My chest, shoulders, back, legs and arms increased in circumference by two-fold. And in a couple more weeks, my pant size shrunk even more, and my muscle mass increased even further…and within 12 weeks, people mistook me for a professional athlete.

In a short period of time, I had accomplished what I couldn't in years.

I have attained my goal physique, and I have shared this program with my gym friends, and colleagues who have accomplished extraordinary results.

How?

I had been painstakingly torturing myself at the gym for years, doing endless cardio, and consuming the most undesired foods, which led to nothing!

Again, the reason is because the information available in the weight loss and bodybuilding community is incomplete or incorrect.

The body building community teaches:

✓ Eat as much protein as possible and pump iron.
(Terrible mistake!)

Consuming large amounts of protein is acid-forming and provides the worst source of fuel. It interrupts the digestive process and clogs the bowels. Protein is the dirtiest source of fuel for the body out of fats, carbohydrates, and proteins. Only enough protein is necessary to repair muscle, which is far less than you might realize.

✓ Eat 4-6 small meals a day. (Terrible mistake!)

Eating 4-6 small meals a day will force the body into a chronic sugar-burning state, which leads to muscle mass deterioration.

What is the logic behind eating 4-6 small meals a day? When did you first learn and apply this approach?

If you do manage to build muscle following the advice from the bodybuilding community, how is muscle mass going to be maintained long term? All the muscle mass that was built over the past weeks, months or years will rapidly deteriorate because the above advice doesn't address how to build or maintain muscle mass in the first place. All the muscle mass that was built over the past weeks, months or years will rapidly deteriorate because the above advice doesn't address how to build or maintain muscle mass.

Bodybuilders who do consume large amounts of protein and eat 4-6 meals a day struggle to maintain muscle mass, and unnecessarily spend hours upon hours at the gym for years because they don't understand what causes muscle mass loss or how to accurately maintain muscle mass.

Only 8 - 10 weeks of intense training is required to attain the physique of your choice. After the 8 – 10 week training session, working out each body part once a week or once every two weeks will suffice for muscle mass to never deteriorate and to maintain a muscular physique permanently.

Bottom line:

How is excess body fat accumulation burnt off without any harmful side effects and a slim physique maintained permanently?

Good question!

I have put together a step-by-step method that will:

1. Burn body fat completely.

2. Maintain a slim physique permanently.

Building a toned and slim physique without compromising or harming the body in any way is what this program is all about.

The results are the bottom line. Burning off body fat completely without compromising or harming the body in any way is what this program is all about.

By applying the methods in this program, you will strengthen your muscles and burn body fat completely and obtain a complete understanding on how to design and control your body in any way you see fit.

The point is this: If you know how your body functions, you can adjust it any way you like.

Like Michelangelo as he sculpted David, from a distance he observed the statue, added a bit more shoulder, chipped away some of the mid-section around the abs, and added more clay on the upper chest.

You are now the Michelangelo of your own body, and you can sculpt a beautiful physique if you learn how to and take action on what you learn.

Think about what happens inside the body to accumulate excess body fat.

Sugar-burning state vs fat-burning state

Think of the body like a vehicle. A vehicle requires a source of fuel to function. If the fuel is dirty or burns out too quickly (protein-burning state or sugar-burning state), the vehicle will not be able to run for long periods of time and will shut down fairly rapidly. In order for the vehicle to function properly for long periods of time, the fuel must be clean, of high quality and burn for hours on end (fat-burning state).

Dishwashing-machine analogy (digestion):

To wash a set of dirty dishes, the rack of the dishwasher must be fully packed with unwashed dishes. The washing process itself takes 30 minutes to complete. Once the wash is done, a new set of dishes are inserted for a new wash session.

Would it make any sense to fill a rack ¼ of the way, begin washing, pause the machine 5 minutes later, fill in another ¼, then wash for another 5 minutes, jam in ¼ then stop everything again and fill in the final ¼?

Hello!?

Four to six small meals a day will force the body into a chronic sugar-burning state, because the body is forcefully trained to burn sugar as opposed to fat. Well this is exactly what is happening to the digestive system if you follow the advice from the bodybuilding community and most weight loss diets.

By eating 2-3 large meals a day, consuming the right saturated fats, avoiding refined carbohydrates/starch and sugars, digestion will function at its peak, blood sugar levels will remain low and fat will be used for fuel.

Where does muscle building and muscle strengthening occur?

✓ What strengthens muscles?

What happens inside the body to build muscles?

Which organs are responsible for building muscle?

The ease of digestion and the digestive effort required for the stomach to digest is what builds muscles.

Amino acids (L-glutamine) are responsible for regenerating muscles after tearing.

Combining the two strategies above will strengthen/tone muscles and burn off existing body fat completely.

Why/how does excess fat accumulate in the body?

✓ What happens inside the body to accumulate excess body fat?

When blood sugar levels spike, the body will use sugar as fuel, which will lead to a chronic sugar-burning state, which leads to accumulation of excess body fat and deterioration of muscle mass.

✓ How is a slim physique maintained after excess body fat has been burnt off?

The body must be in a chronic fat-burning state.

Toning/strengthening the muscles occurs during digestion.

If digestion is strong+ fast + easy = building muscles will be strong + fast + easy.

Weight loss vs bodybuilding:

My story leans more towards bodybuilding. However, the basic principles are the same. Weight training is necessary to burn body fat. Contrary to popular belief, walking, cycling, or jogging (cardio) alone will not burn body fat completely.

More than 95% of body fat is burnt off by strengthening/toning muscle fibers of the body.

Note: Toning/strengthening the muscles is NOT the same as building muscle mass.

Building large muscle mass for bodybuilders is hard.

Strengthening the muscles to lose weight is easy.

Does this sound different then what you are used to?

Does it seem like a new way to trim fat?

Are you confused?

If you answered yes to all the above...

Don't worry.

In this program, everything you need to know is covered in detail.

And I assure you that you will experience results.

What about existing body fat?

Strengthening the muscles by lifting weights and avoiding/replacing fattening foods with non-fattening foods will burn off body fat completely. In addition, proper doses of amino acids further burn body fat and repairs/regenerates muscle mass.

You must know which foods cause body fat to accumulate and replace those foods with non-fattening foods. This does not mean cutting out all carbohydrates; some carbohydrates are necessary since they are nutrient dense.

Basics:

As food is chewed, food particles are fully digested in the stomach and in the small and large intestines. Food nutrients are absorbed in the intestinal wall. Then the nutrient-packed blood circulates throughout the body into each individual cell. Whatever particles remain or are left over from digestion turn to waste and are expelled by the bowels (excretion).

If food is burdensome to digest, the bowels will become sluggish, acidic and congested. All the nutrients absorbed by the intestinal walls and stomach walls will be severely compromised.

Digestion occurs in the stomach.

Pathways of elimination:

The entire human body is a compact system of tubes. The veins, bowels, muscles, and individual cells are only a bunch of tubes. If the tubes become congested or blocked, toxicity will build up over time.

The body expels waste through the bowels, kidneys, skin and lungs. If the bowels (primary pathway of elimination) become overloaded, the body is forced to pack away fat tissue.

If the bowels become clogged or blocked for long periods of time, waste is expelled through the skin and lungs (secondary pathways of elimination).

Note: The ideal place to begin is by doing a deep internal detoxification cleanse. The cleanse will get rid of unnecessary gunk in the bowels, unclogging the internal tubes.

What does this mean?

Digestion and assimilation have to be strong. The system has to be clean and old waste must be eliminated from the system quickly.

Sum it all up:

The principles in this program are very powerful, and most of them are simple.

You might ask: But isn't everyone's body different?

Answer: Everyone's body, internal organs, digestion, elimination, and assimilation function are *exactly the same*.

However, you must have an open mind and commit to this program for 8 - 10 weeks to see the results you are after.

Have faith in the program and it will work and you will succeed.

You must let go of the old beliefs from years prior, and set out a new path.

If you keep doing everything the same, you will never achieve any kind of new results!

This program will not place you in the top 5% of fitness enthusiasts, weight loss gurus, or whoever else at the gym—it will place you in the top 1%.

Steps:

1. What to eat

2. Supplements to take

3. How to fire up digestion

4. Transplant friendly bacteria

Step 1 prevents any further fat accumulation, supports digestion, helps bowels to be free of waste, and keeps the system clean. Steps 2, 3 and 4 strengthen the muscles, prevent the muscles from deterioration and burn body fat.

None of the steps are theories or guesswork.

All the steps have been tested, and you will see results.

Ordinary or average results, or experiencing zero results is a thing of the past. And of course, this program delivers **long-lasting** results.

Our body is the most precious gift we have. But the body doesn't come with a manual at birth. Here is some basic knowledge required to strengthen muscles, burn all body fat and maintain a slim physique permanently.

A lot of information? Yes…you will have to read this text more than once to fully understand how weight loss really works.

In this step-by-step program, you will learn how to perfect everything mentioned above.

Before we move on…

Let me make one thing absolutely clear from the start:

I am not interested in advertising supplements,

nor am I pushing anyone to buy supplements.

Some or most of the nutrients listed here have to be taken externally. Meaning our bodies cannot produce them on its own. From foods alone, nutrients are impossible to be absorbed.

My only interest is for you to achieve your health/fitness goals after having come across my program.

This program is means serious business, and only those who are dedicated can follow.

Back to business…

It is possible that you can be overwhelmed by the quantity of supplements in this program. 60% of the supplements are absolutely necessary for weight loss, and 40% are not absolutely necessary.

Absolutely necessary: **coconut oil, green drinks, L-glutamine, probiotics and inulin.**

Not absolutely necessary: flavored stevia, fiber, magnesium, flax oil, cod liver oil and calcium.

The necessary supplements add up to $90 - $150. The additional supplements have been added to make my reader's life more pleasurable and for you to have a more complete understanding of the information in this program and what the human body requires.

If you find yourself still complaining about spending $90 - $150 on the necessary supplements, look at the program this way. Most fitness, workout, and weight loss programs costs $150+ for the information alone. In addition, those programs recommend chemically bastardized supplements that carry harmful side effects, such as whey protein, hydroxycut, creatine, etc. And 9/10 weight loss or fitness programs available deliver zero results.

The supplements listed in this program are all NATURAL and do not carry any harmful side effects whatsoever. Don't believe anything you read here; look up side effects of hydroxycut. Believe me, this is not the path to lose weight. The necessary supplements are not listed in these pages just for curiosity sake. Each and every one has been tested, which led to maximize results of bodybuilding, weight loss and maintaining muscle mass.

I wish there was a magic pill that would automatically build muscles and burn fat without any diet or exercise, but this isn't reality! The reality is that building muscle mass requires effort, persistence, dietary changes and money on the part of the participant.

If you still can't agree to spend at least $150 on the necessary supplements…**stop reading right now!** Because this program is not for you.

Read and study each of the supplements. Choose one from each category that best suits your taste and goals.

BONUS #1:

On the bonus chapter labeled "Workout," you will find the workout routine that is most effective for building muscle mass and burning body fat.

BONUS #2:

At the end of the book, you will find a link that leads to a squeeze page where you can, and absolutely should, enter your email address for future health and fitness products from me.

I'm won't mail out weekly updates—none of that nonsense. I'm going to mail out only crucial information and products that I personally use relevant to fitness and health.

This program only covers the basics on weight loss.

There is also a lot of information I just couldn't cram into this short book. If you apply the methods in this program and experience outstanding results (which you will), sign up for future notices.

Let's begin with step 1…

Step 1: WHAT TO EAT

Protein clarified:

Out of carbohydrates, fats, and protein, protein is by far the worst source of fuel for the human body. After the protein is burned as fuel, debris is left behind known as ketones, which cause acidic buildup within the system. Small amounts of protein should be ingested and kept in balance with cleansing foods.

The information on how much protein an average non-athletic to athletic type individual should consume drastically differs from health experts to health magazines to the bodybuilding community and weight loss community.

There are too many factors to consider depending on how much the muscles are torn during workouts, if the body is growing into adulthood, etc. This is why following one protein regimen isn't ideal.

However, the average diet alone is already packed with more than enough protein than necessary.

Questions:

- Why do you _**believe**_ large doses of protein are needed for bodybuilding or weight loss?
- Can you pinpoint how protein builds muscle or burns body fat?
- Where did you first buy into this idea?

On the topic of beliefs....

Question all your beliefs.

Question where your beliefs came from.

What are beliefs?

Beliefs are cause and effect equations.

Beliefs are a patterned system of perspectives.

Physical reality can be compared to a mirror; what we believe most strongly to be true, is true. A mirror can only reflect. If you believe in the definition "no pain - no gain," then you will be unable to experience any gains without pain. But the truth is that you can experience gains without any pain.

Actually, a few members have reported that they only feel the pump, and not the painful recovery, and you can too.

I believe that if I do such and such, the result will be such and such, and so it does.

If A happens, B will follow.

A and B can be any definition you wish.

For example if you believe

"Success = A and difficulty = B," then this belief will result in experiencing hardships and struggles in your life, and you will only attract and experience un-successful circumstances and success will always be hard to reach.

If you believe "Success is effortless," life will be a spectacular experience. You can only attract successful circumstance and situations.

For example, if you believe "I am unattractive to the opposite gender" or "Getting in shape is hard" or "Life is hard," where did these beliefs come from? Parents? Society? Friends? and when... during kindergarten? elementary or middle school?

Most everyone on this planet is dragging along beliefs that do not belong to themselves. That is why out body feels so heavy. Identify where all your negative or unnecessary beliefs came from. Once the belief has been identified, like placing a spotlight on a burglar escaping from prison, the belief will disappear.

The negative belief will appear to be nonsensical and illogical to continue to carry. You will realize that the belief your holding onto came from an external source… and now you can simply delete the old, useless belief, and replace with new definitions.

Simply re-define all your unnecessary beliefs with a new definition,

"Success is difficult,"

to

"Success is easy and effortless."

Back to business.

Just taking in as much protein will do nothing but cause damage in the long run.

Think about what happens inside the body to build muscle and burn fat.

Most likely you have been consuming protein powder, chicken breasts, and beef…and you still haven't seen any results, which is why you are reading this book!

Buying into the protein diet is a perfect example of the blind leading the blind. If you don't want to belong to the bottom 95%, you have to stop conforming to these ideas right now!

Keep in mind the vehicle analogy. If large amounts of protein are consumed in excess, the body will use protein as fuel— **WHICH IS THE SOURCE OF FUEL TO AVOID**.

Stay with me here.

A large majority of professional athletes, fitness models and bodybuilders go through a whole lot of trouble to obtain illegal substances, such as steroids, testosterone, or they inject oils directly into their bodies, which eventually gets them expelled from their professions, develop disease, have incontrollable tempers, and in extreme cases an early death.

If the protein path works, why do these professionals consume illegal steroids? The reason is because eating 4-6 small meals a day coupled with large doses of protein only delivers temporary, short-lived results and causes harmful side effects in the long run.

Research pro-athletes from the 70s, 80s and 90s. If they aren't dead already, they most likely are suffering from heart enlargement, liver disease, bloating of the bowels, and female athletes who consumed testosterone now look like men and they have an entire list of health problems you don't want to ever deal with.

Life shouldn't be full of struggle. Weight loss is not hard. Body fat can be burnt off completely and naturally without any kind of harmful side effects.

Believe me, I took large amounts of protein for years. I'm sure you know what I'm talking about. What you are getting from me is direct experience on myself and others.

You have to follow through in your best judgment with the teachings in this text to 8 - 10 weeks, and experience the results yourself.

Let me repeat one last time:

The truth is that most meals are already loaded with more proteins than necessary. Whole grains, vegetables and fruits are packed with way more protein than the body requires.

Protein facts (from USDA: United States Department of Agriculture):

Nutrients: Protein (g)

Measured by: 100 g protein (g) value per

Vegetables:

Garlic, raw – 6.36g

Kale, raw – 4.28g

Spinach, raw – 2.86g

Onions, sweet, raw – 0.80

Broccoli raab, raw – 3.17g

Kale, frozen, unprepared – 2.66g

Edamame, frozen, unprepared – 11.32g

Nuts and seeds:

Nuts, almond butter, plain – 20.96g

Nuts, chestnuts, Chinese, dried – 6.82g

Soybeans, green, cooked, boiled, drained – 12.35g

Beans, kidney, mature seeds, sprouted, raw – 4.20g

Beans, pinto, immature seeds, frozen, unprepared– 9.80g

Nuts, cashew butter, plain, without salt added – 17.56g

Cooked vegetables and baked foods:

Potatoes, baked, skin – 4.29g

Peppers, sweet, green, dried – 17.90g
Mushrooms, portabella, grilled – 3.28g

Peas and carrots, frozen, cooked, boiled, drained – 3.09g

Potatoes, mashed, dehydrated, flakes without milk, dry form – 8.38g

Bagels, wheat – 10.20g

Bread, egg, toasted – 10.20g

Bread, Boston brown, canned – 5.20g

Homestyle cookies, sugar-free oatmeal – 5.54g

Protein becomes difficult to digest in the system if consumed in large quantities or excess. High protein foods must be consumed in moderate quantities combined with cleansing foods for ease of digestion. The only people who should be consuming large amounts of protein are small children still growing into adulthood.

Sugars and refined starch:

Think of sugars as a source of fuel.

Refined starch: refined flour, white flour, and white grains have the same effect as sugar.

When sugar is consumed, sugar travels up the bloodstream violently spiking blood sugar levels like nothing else. The body is forced to lower the blood sugar levels rapidly. The body releases a strong rush of insulin to force the blood sugar levels into body's sugar depository, the muscles and liver. White sugar is completely incompatible to the human body, causing disease and body fat.

Sugars and refined starches don't have any place in your diet during and after the completion of this program.

Analogy of a sink:

Water = sugar

Pressure of water from the faucet = amount of sugar consumed at one time.

Water (sugar) pours into the sink (body) from the faucet, and the water is expelled down the drain (sugar burnt by metabolic rate). The pressure or force of the running water depends on how much sugar is consumed at a time. The more sugar, the more powerful the pressure will be.

What happens if water pours down faster than the drain is able to expel? Eventually, the sink will overflow and spill over, become excess body fat, and kick the body into a sugar-burning state.

The analogy of the sink can be compared to the body's sugar depository, which comes down to the muscle mass and the liver. If the sink spills over from consuming too much sugar at one time, the body will be forced to burn the sugar as its source of fuel.

What will happen if the body is already packed with sugar?

The body will be forced to:

1. Eliminate sugar through the kidneys or urine.

2. The liver converts the sugar into lard, which is stored as body fat to be used as energy.

If the sink (body) overflows, then muscle mass will be lost and excess body fat gained.

The essential point of the sink analogy is to avoid eating large amounts of sugar/refined starch/refined carbohydrates at any one time.

Healthy sugars: Natural sweeteners like raw honey, maple syrup, fruits, and black strap molasses are healthy sugars that provide nutrients for the body.

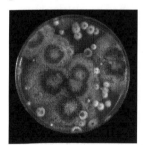

Note: Even healthy sugars and fructose in fruits shouldn't be consumed in large quantities at any one time, or else blood sugars will spike just like with refined sugars.

Fruits are loaded with fiber, but they are also loaded with natural sugars. These natural sugars not only spike blood insulin levels but can cause fungal, mold and candida overgrowth. Consume only a handful of fruits at a time.

Fruit juices are packed with fructose. Apart from lime juice, avoiding fruit juices completely during the duration of the program is ideal.

Unhealthy sugars: Refined and processed sugars, cane sugar, aspartame, fructose corn syrup, saccharine, and NutraSweet only cause body fat to accumulate, don't carry any nutrients, and destroy nutrients in the body.

Carbohydrates and starch divided into 4 groups:

Simple: honey, maple syrup, molasses

Refined: white sugar, white rice, refined fours

Complex: whole grains, whole starch, potatoes

Complex and fiber rich: sprouts and vegetables

Refined carbohydrates cause severe spikes of blood sugar levels, increased body fat, and loss of muscle mass. They do nothing positive to the body and cause disease and damage to health.

Grains, sugars and starches are very acid-forming inside the system. Once converted into simple sugars, the body will use grains, sugars and starch as its source of fuel (sugar-burning state).

Complex fiber, rich raw vegetables and highly alkalizing foods like sprouts and green vegetables are cleansing. The more amounts of raw vegetables and green drinks consumed the healthier, more alkaline you will be.

Complex whole grains, potatoes, etc. must be balanced with cleansing foods (cleansing foods 2/3 vs solid foods 1/3).

Simple carbohydrates, starch and fructose must also be kept to a minimum.

What to avoid (refined):

- Pastries
- Junk food (chocolate, candy, etc.)
- Soft drinks
- White flour, refined pasta

- White flour, refined bread
- High fructose syrup

Refined carbohydrates will only cause excess body fat accumulation and eat away all the nutrients from the body. Refined carbohydrates don't carry any benefits whatsoever. It would be wise to cut out refined carbohydrates completely during the 10-12 weeks of the program.

Solution to sweets:

Omitting sweets completely can make a person go crazy. I especially love sweetened hot cocoa!

What if there is a way to sweeten all drinks and foods and not have blood sugars spike or kick the body into a sugar-burning state whatsoever?

Luckily, there is a simple yet effective way that can replace sugar in all foods and drinks.

The perfect replacement for sugar:

Stevia is several hundred times sweeter than sugar and will never spike blood sugar levels. The most overweight person in the world can consume an unlimited amount of stevia and they will never gain an ounce of body fat. But remember to not add too much because of its extreme sweetness.

All natural supplements are listed in:

www.nekoterran.com/supplements

Choose only one supplement from each category.

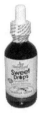

Wisdom Natural, SweetLeaf Liquid Stevia, Sweet Drops Sweetener, Vanilla I,
2 fl oz (60 ml) $9.21

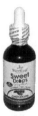

Wisdom Natural, SweetLeaf Liquid Stevia, Sweet Drops Sweetener, Chocolate,
2 fl oz (60 ml) $9.58

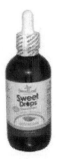

Sweet Leaf Liquid Stevia, Clear, 120 ml, 4 oz $20.41

These are my favorite stevia extract liquid products. I love to mix vanilla stevia with my green drinks and in my occasional hot cocoa. Green drinks are absolutely crucial to optimal health, but they aren't the best-tasting drinks. Stevia can be added pretty much anywhere—in cooked food, as salad dressing, mixed with coconut oil…be creative and experiment with what works best for you.

Don't be afraid to try different stevia products. Stevia plants are absolutely safe and from nature. Find the right flavor and taste for each of your drinks and foods.

Note: The stevia products above DO NOT contain inulin or FOS.

Inulin is the special fiber that feeds on friendly bacteria to prosper in the intestines. In the transplant-friendly bacteria chapter, specific inulin stevia extracts are recommended.

Refined grains:

Rice and flour, after refinement, turn into nutrition-less food packed with starch junk that will harden into mucoid plaque in the stomach and intestinal walls when consumed. Refined grains and flour clog the system, causing stress on digestion.

Large amounts of starch, grains and sugars provoke severe acid buildup in the system.

If too much starch, refined carbohydrates or sugars is consumed at any one time, the system will flood and spill over.

The only kinds of rice that should be ingested are whole grain brown rice and whole grain wild rice. This rice won't cause acid build up or congest the system if consumed together with cleansing foods. Solid or building-food intake should make up 1/3 of your overall diet. Be sure to eat whole grains and wild grains balanced with cleansing foods that should make up 2/3 of overall food intake.

Starchy vegetables:

Starchy vegetables include white potatoes, red potatoes, sweet potatoes, pumpkin, zucchini, yams, onion, beets, carrots, celery root and root type vegetables. Starchy vegetables taste better cooked. Cooking starchy vegetables reduces the starch content within these vegetables, making them easier to digest.

Non-starchy vegetables:

The very best source of carbohydrates are non-starchy vegetables. Non-starchy vegetables are the best to juice and should make up the majority of your diet. These vegetables are full of fiber and enzymes and are easiest to digest. Some examples would include cabbage, lettuce, broccoli, cucumber, tomatoes and sprouts. Anything green and leafy would be categorized as a non-starchy vegetable.

Solid foods vs cleansing foods:

Foods react individually inside the body. Some foods cleanse the system, and other foods build. The body needs a balance of both. Solid foods alone will cause blockages in the system, acid buildup and constipation. Eating only cleansing foods will lead to nutrient deficiencies.

The balance of the two is key. Raw green vegetables are very easy to digest, create an alkaline environment within the system, and make bowel transit fast and easy.

Solid foods, also known as building foods, have the opposite effect.

Solid foods: Should make up 1/3 of over food intake.

- Cooked vegetables
- Meat (chicken, fish)
- Wild, brown rice
- Wild, brown bread
- Beans and lentils

- Whole bread
- Whole grains
- Eggs
- Starchy vegetables

Cleansing foods: Make up 2/3 of overall food intake.

- Raw non-starchy vegetables.
- Anything green, leafy and raw plant-based
- Green drinks
- Fruits and fruit juices (keep in mind fructose sugars, sink analogy)

Alkaline:

al·ka·line

having the properties of an alkali; having a pH greater than 7.

The body's blood levels must have pH levels greater than 7. An alkaline environment in the bowels prevents acid buildup and is absolutely essential to strengthen the muscles, burn body fat, and achieve optimal health. An acidic environment invites parasites, molds and fungal overgrowth. The more amounts of green drinks, raw vegetables, and sprouts you intake, the better. The more physical activity you are involved in, the more alkaline your system needs to be.

The overall food intake of 2/3 cleansing foods and 1/3 solid foods may clash with what you are used to, and demanding in the beginning, but if you are serious about getting in top shape, dietary changes must be made.

Remember that digestion must be strong, easy and quick to build muscle mass.

The solution is to create an alkaline environment within, which allows intestinal flora (friendly bacteria) to flourish and prevents unfriendly bacteria overgrowth and other intestinal problems. To create an alkaline environment, eating solid raw vegetables alone is insufficient. The bulk of food intake should be green vegetables. In addition, juicing vegetables or green drinks are necessary to achieve an alkaline internal environment.

What are green drinks?

Green drink is another name for vegetable juice and grass juice.

Any non-starchy vegetables are great to juice with a pinch of lime or stevia to improve the taste.

How many lemons have to be squeezed for one drinking glass? 5-6 lemons or more?

The point is, by juicing vegetables, large quantities of vegetables that cannot possibly be consumed in solid form can be consumed in juice form. Never underestimate the power of juicing. A highly alkaline internal environment will boost energy and maintain a clean internal system.

Alkaline body pH levels, the internal environment established inside the intestines, is crucial for health, internal detoxification, weight loss, bodybuilding...everything! If you keep your vehicle (body) clean→ disease, body fat, loss of muscle, aging process (oxidation), mucoid plaque, parasites, molds, candida and fungal overgrowth cannot survive. Have alkaline pH levels cannot be emphasized enough. And of course, a deep internal detoxification will go a long way in keeping the system clean.

Purchasing a quality blender can be a life-changing event. Juicing green drinks or juicing anything else and pretty much cooking overall will never be the same experience from this point onwards.

Most cheap blenders break down, burn out, and over heat the vegetable juices. As you will learn, if the vegetable juices are heated, enzymes within the raw plants will die.

Choose a blender of your choice.

FREE shipping.

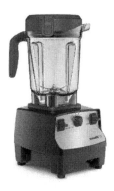

Certified Reconditioned- 5300 $299

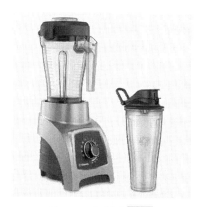

Personal- S30 $329

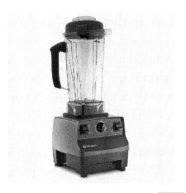

Legacy (food blender) - 5200 $449

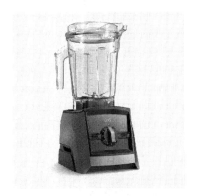

Ascent Series A2300 $469

Some chain names that use Vitamix:

Starbucks, Beans Bins, Jamba Juice, Jugo Juice, Booster Juice, Lavazza Coffee, Tully's, Costa Coffee, Robeks, Maui Wowi Hawaiian Coffee & Smoothies, Smoothie King, Mr.

Smoothie, Orange Julius, Tropical Smoothie Café, and the list goes on.

The next time you visit any coffee, juice, or smoothie chain store, sneak a peek at what blender they are using. I assure you they will be using a Vitamix blender...and there is a reason for this.

The reason is because Vitamix blenders are of the highest quality, incomparable to any other blender in the marketplace.

The feature I like the most about the Vitamix blender is that the motor is extremely powerful and will never overheat the vegetable juices, keeping the enzymes alive. The only downside I can think of is that the motor is loud and heavy.

All the recipes available at the chain names can be replicated at home using the Vitamix blender. Even healthy alternatives for ice-cream, junk foods, chocolate shakes, sauces, dressings, and even soups can be made. Any kind of unhealthy food or sugar-packed junk food has a healthy substitute using a high-quality blender. Believe me, cooking will never be the same again.

To juice using a blender or juicer is the traditional way of juicing. This approach requires a high-quality blender and large amounts of vegetables, and it is extremely time consuming. Any green leafy non-starchy vegetable would be ok to juice, including seaweed. This method is the best; however, the downside of using a juicer is that it can be expensive. If you are able to juice vegetables, that would be the number one choice.

The good news: There is a cheaper yet effective way to consume alkalizing vegetable drinks, and that is with green drink powder. Green drink powders are the fast food replacement for juicing vegetables.

Here are some of my favorite products that taste delicious combined with flavored or inulin stevia.

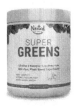

SUPER GREENS, #1 Green Veggie Superfood Powder, 8.5 oz $24.95

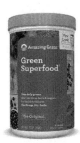

Amazing Grass Green Superfood, Original, Powder, 60 servings $33.55

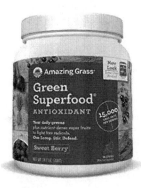

Amazing Grass Green SuperFood ORAC, 100 Servings, 24.7 oz $48.39

The bulk of alkalizing green nutrition in these supplements does not differ so much. On the other hand, the taste differs drastically with each product. I like to swap products once in a while. Read the nutritional label and ingredients section of each green powder before ordering.

Acidity: the enemy of alkaline

Acidity is the opposite of alkaline.

Acidic blood pollutes the bowels like nothing else. 'Acidosis' is the name for high levels of acid build up in the system. Many of the health consequences people suffer from is directly linked to our diets. And acidosis is one of the worst. Tumors are a good example. A tumor grows/lives/multiplies in acidic environments.

Blood Cells

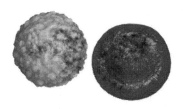

When you observe nature and evolution, notice that fish grow fins, scaly skin and gills to adapt to oceans and rivers. Carnivores, like mountain lions, grow large fangs and claws to hunt their prey. Frogs develop webs between their fingers to swim, etc. Lifeforms morph, mutate and transform according to their corresponding environment.

Inside our bodies, red blood cells will actually morph into dangerous antibodies to adapt to the acidic/polluted environment that causes disease.

Healthy Blood Cells

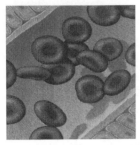

The same rule applies when the internal system is clean/alkaline. Molds, parasites, internal pollution and disease cannot survive. An acidic internal environment also leads to unfriendly bacteria overgrowth, which can destroy friendly bacteria transplanted in the bowels.

Let me repeat:

The internal ENVIRONMENT of the body is what makes the difference between an acidic system and an alkaline system.

Primary causes of acid buildup in the system:

1. Solid foods unbalanced with cleansing foods.

2. Poor digestion. If food isn't properly digested, undigested food particles will cause acid buildup in the bowels.

3. Acid forming foods and drinks.

Certain foods cause acid buildup, and others are alkaline producing. Consuming some acid-forming foods is ok and necessary, but the majority of food intake should consist of raw vegetables and green drinks (cleansing foods). By controlling the consumption of congesting foods with alkalizing foods/drinks, the system will remain at an alkaline level.

Alkalinity is absolutely crucial to achieve a healthy, fat free and fit physique.

Acid-forming foods that have to be kept to a minimum or cut out during the 12 weeks:

• Refined grains

- Sugars and refined starch

- Protein powder

- Protein in excess

- Cooked food in excess not balance with cleansing foods

- Cow milk

Cow Milk:

Milk in its natural form is raw milk,' and it is put in the category of alkaline drinks. The milk 99% of people drink, bought from the supermarket that has been pasteurized and homogenized becomes acidic.

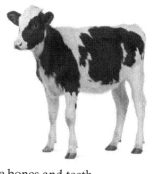

The advertisement industry has persuaded the general public to believe that cow milk, and dairy products from cows strengthens the bones and teeth.

Is cow milk really beneficial for us humans?

What is the evidence?

Contrary to popular belief, all foods from cow milk are the most blood polluting, system clogging, acid forming, blood dirtying, mucoid plaque forming, allergy inducing foods available.

Cow milk is extremely high in caseinate, which is strenuous to digest. Not only this, the health industry demands all cow milk to go through the process of pasteurization to kill bacteria. Pasteurization will wipe out protein, fats and all benefits of cow milk.

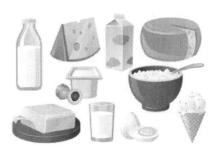

Whey protein and casein protein consumed by the bodybuilding and health communities are some of the worst. Pasteurized, conventional cow milk causes blood cells to become congested by toxins, accumulates mucoid plaque due to the disease and allergies dairy causes.

Drinking whey protein shakes, casein protein, or just plain cow milk is equivalent to ingesting clay that will harden inside the stomach and intestinal walls. Mucoid plaque buildup will severely clog the system.

You've probably been programmed that cow milk is one of the necessary food groups that provides calcium. On the contrary, this is so far from the truth.

Evidence:

North America, Canada, UK, and a few European countries are the Western territories that consume the most cow milk in the world. They are also the countries that have the highest numbers of osteoporosis sufferers.

Vice versa, a child born and raised in Asia or in the tropical equator, is far less likely to ever suffer from osteoporosis, or any other diseases related to the bones, compared to a child growing up in the US or Europe.

Mayo Clinic definition:

Osteoporosis:

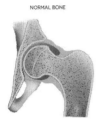 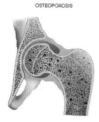

Osteoporosis causes bones to become weak and brittle—so brittle that a fall or even mild stresses like bending over or coughing can cause a fracture. Osteoporosis-related fractures most commonly occur in the hip, wrist or spine.

Cow milk is extremely high in protein and phosphorous. Large doses of protein cause tissues to become acidic.

The human body must maintain a pH level between 7.35 and 7.45 for the body to survive. A pH level below 6.8 or above 7.8 will viciously morph the cells in the body, which leads to illness, and eventually death. Our bodies are designed by nature to maintain slight alkaline pH levels to live.

What does this mean?

Processed, refined foods, cow milk and processed oils we consume creates a highly acidic internal environment within. The body will forcibly counterbalance the acidity to maintain a slight alkaline system to survive.

If diet doesn't support alkalinity, the body will be forced to leach out to other places in the body, like the bones to maintain proper pH levels. Over the period of years of consuming the wrong foods, the bones will be stripped away from, or 'hit' on a regular basis, leading to weakness, frailness, fractures, and osteoporosis (more on cow milk section).

When consuming whey protein powder or cow milk in excess, the bones actually deteriorate.

More evidence:

Humans have been programmed since childhood to drink cow milk. Cow milk is by nature tailored for a baby calf to grow from 40kg (90 pounds) at birth to 700kg (1,500 pounds) in only two years. Cows have four stomachs, and their digestive systems function nothing like a human's. The casein found in cow milk simply can't be adaptable by humans.

And we are supposed to drink cow milk for health reasons. What kind of crazy logic is this?

All dairy products, casein and whey protein must be cut out altogether, unless you choose to suffer from the above.

Red Meat

The IARC (International Agency of Research on Cancer) labels the following as "red meat":

- beef
- veal
- pork
- lamb
- mutton
- horse
- goat

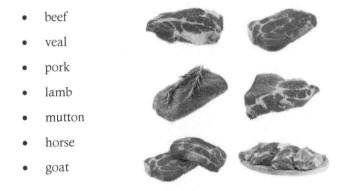

Red meat is the most burdensome mammal meat to digest. In almost all cases, red meat leads to poor digestion, partial digestion, and acid buildup in the bowels. A more serious problem would be partially digested foods actually rots within the bowels. Chronic consumption of red meat will congest and clog the bowels due to mucoid plaque buildup. Like snot forming in the nostrils, mucoid plaque is a protective mechanism the body discharges to protect the internal organs. The more incompatible foods inserted into the system, the more mucoid plaque will form, which leads to constipation.

When eating mammal meat, more cleansing raw vegetables have to be consumed for more emphasis to be put on digestion.

Although I am not a fan of eating any kind of animal meat, a better replacement for red meat would be fish or bird meat like turkey.

Fried foods

When oil is heated, it becomes an unstable militant. Heated oils morph into toxic waste—an acid-forming substance that destroys all fats, carbohydrates, friendly bacteria, protein and everything it comes in contact with. Fried foods, or heated oils, could be said to lead the body into a "**toxic** sugar-burning state," which is far worse than a normal sugar-burning state alone. Foods deep fried in vegetable oils are the most fattening, muscle mass deteriorating foods you can possibly ingest. Vegetable cooking oils used cause the most damage to the liver and intestinal walls. Most vegetable oils go through the process of hydrogenation.

A great example would be McDonald's. McDonald's burgers actually aren't very fattening. What is causing all the health problems and fat accumulation are the deep-fried French fries and chicken nuggets. Even the healthiest foods become toxic once fried in vegetable oil.

Although every kind of fried oil is not recommended, if fried food must be consumed, the best oil to use is unrefined coconut oil for cooking.

If you absolutely must consume fried food, cooking with coconut oil is the answer. Saturated fats found in unrefined coconut oils are less toxic and far more stable when heated compared to vegetable oils. But keep in mind that all fried food is best kept to a minimum or avoided all together.

What to eat in summary:

Counting calories and measuring foods in grams complicates everything and makes weight loss and bodybuilding an un-desired process. Raw vegetables, green drinks and keeping blood insulin levels low will never cause body fat or deteriorate muscle mass.

Use your common sense!

If you don't eat anything fattening and keep your system clean, you will never become fat!

The greener, the better:

- Alkaline foods should make up more than half to 2/3 of your overall food intake.

- Consume highly alkalizing green drinks and grass/green juices.

- Fill up on cleansing raw vegetables.

All cooked foods, be it cooked vegetables, cooked meat, cooked whole grains, should make up 1/3 of your total intake. Consume fruits in small portions due to high fructose content.

Supplements:

Take 6 or more tablespoons of coconut oil a day.

Take 6 or more caplets of probiotics in the morning or before going to sleep in an empty stomach.

Absolutely necessary: coconut oil, green drinks, L-glutamine, probiotics and inulin.

Not absolutely necessary: flavored stevia, fiber, magnesium, cod liver oil, flax oil and calcium.

Directions for green drinks... Per Drinking Glass:

1 teaspoon of green powder + mix a tablespoon of fiber

+ inulin stevia + 1 teaspoon of L-glutamine

in a glass of water x3 times a day.

Foods to avoid and what to replace with:

<u>Avoid</u> →	<u>Replace with</u>
Sugars (refined)	Stevia extract
White flour, white rice (refined carbs)......	Whole grains, wild rice, brown bread
Deep fried food (eg. French fries)............	Baked food (baked potato)
Cow milk, dairy foods	Calcium and magnesium
Hydrogenated Vegetable oil, cooking oil...	Unrefined coconut oil
Red meat (beef, pork)	Fish, turkey, chicken, bird meat

Eat 1 or more eggs a day (cholesterol).

By avoiding and replacing the foods mentioned above, you are well on your way to building a fat-less, muscular physique.

More on What to Eat:

After all the diet/nutrition facts has been laid out in detail, I'm still bombarded with emails asking....

- *What do I eat?*

- *What protein powder should I take?*

- *How much protein should I take?*

- *Is a gram of protein per body pound a day the correct amount?*

- *What about creatine?*

- *What do I eat for breakfast, lunch and dinner?*

- *Coconut oil makes me gag; is there a replacement?*

- *What do I take to boost energy levels?*

- ***What do I eat?***

Remember the rules. If your goal is to get in top shape, diet plays a major role.

70%+ should be easy to digest, raw vegetables, green drinks and water. Only 30% of your overall food intake should be cooked food. Avoid fattening foods, foods that damage the body and clogs the body.

Drink enough water until your urine is clear, as opposed to yellow.

Listen to your body; it gives feedback 24/7.

Of course, eating cookie and cream ice cream topped by melted chocolate will taste better than eating a bunch of raw vegetables. Eating the best tasting foods, is far from listening to your body. By listening to your body, I mean listen to how your body responds to the foods you take in.

Likewise, eating super healthy 24/7 sometimes seems inhuman to do. Most definitely, once in a while you're going to break down and crave junk food. The good news is that there is a heathy alternative to ALL junk foods. By all, I seriously mean all. A super-blender can make hot chocolate, chocolate ice cream, cookie and cream ice cream, muffins, brownies and pretty much can make any sugary food, and most cooked food substitute you can think of.

That is why the Vitamix blender is placed at the top. Super-blenders are an absolute must for green drinks, fitness and every other area in the kitchen. Truly life changing, I highly recommend a quality blender for long-term results.

How to listen to your body:

For example...

If eating cheese (cow milk), pork, beef, deep fried shrimp and nuts make you feel sick, then cut out those foods from your diet. Growing up, I never had a meal that did not have some kind of animal meat. The reality of eating a meal without meat was just beyond the bounds of possibility.

Now the scent of raw meat is intolerable to me. When I do eat any kind of red meat, I can feel the meat rot and putrefy inside my body as it digests. Thirty minutes after the meal, I latch onto my mid-section until the irritation passes.

I don't understand why anyone would eat any kind of animal meat. However, if eating animal meat feels wonderful, by all means, keep animal meat in your diet.

- *What protein powder should I take?*

- *How much protein should I take?*

- *Is a gram of protein per body pound a day the correct amount?*

Avoid any kind of protein shake and avoid increasing the amount of protein intake in your diet. Your diet is already fully packed with more protein than necessary.

When protein is eaten in the correct amount to supply the body with the right amount of amino acids, the body is able to repair its tissues. More protein won't provide more energy; instead, the body has to store/convert the extra protein elsewhere.

- *What about creatine?*

Creatine is an amino acid-**like** substance stored in our muscles as creatine phosphate.

The theory is…

Due to creatine retaining water, some athletes determine that because creatine pulls more water into the muscles, muscles look bigger.

Athletes take creatine to achieve bursts of strength, or to do some extra reps. The other main reason is because creatine is one of the cheaper supplements.

To be totally honest, I have experimented with doses of creatine and saw zero results.

There have been plenty of studies on creatine for the short-term, but still few answers remain for the long-term. There are too many uncertainties with creatine, and enough side effects reported to stay away from the supplement all together.

(Creatine - Mayo Clinic)

- Mild asthma-like symptoms
- high blood pressure
- abnormal heart rate
- Heat intolerance
- Fever
- Dehydration
- reduced blood volume
- electrolyte imbalances (leading to seizures)
- Creatine may turn to creatinine once ingested in the stomach (read The Danger of Creatinine, by Jeff Golini)
- Increase aggressiveness

- Hair loss
- Diarrhea
- Upset stomach
- Muscle cramps
- Dizziness
- Kidney damage
- Liver dysfunction

- ***What do I eat for breakfast, lunch and dinner?***

Cleansing cycle: 5:00 am to 10:00 am (early morning)

Absorption cycle: 10:00 am to 7:00 pm (mid-afternoon)

Assimilation cycle: 7:00 pm to 11 pm (evening

More on the body's natural cycles coming up.

- ***Coconut oil makes me gag; is there a replacement?***

Taste comes last in body building and weight loss. If your goal is to belong to the top 1% - 5%, then you have to follow a path that 99% won't.

Coconut oil prevents the body from going into starvation mode.

What causes hunger?

In most if not all cases, hunger is caused by high and low spikes of blood sugar levels.

Coconut oil stabilizes blood sugar levels immensely. Many days, I would go eating only one meal a day, and I didn't feel any hunger whatsoever. You will know what I mean.

- ***What do I take to boost energy levels?***

When drinking a glass of fresh vegetable or grass juice (green drinks), I can feel my energy levels soaring as the green liquid travels down into my bowels, revitalizing my body to be ready to pump some iron.

Green drinks, coconut oil, right fats and an alkaline diet will boost energy levels more than energizing drinks like Red Bull, black coffee, creatine or any kind or temporary energy booster ever will.

STEP 2. WHAT SUPPLEMENTS TO TAKE

What is eaten doesn't strengthen/tone the muscles. The digestive effort for the stomach to digest is what strengthens muscles.

However, diet plays a critical role. Diet is responsible for digestion to be effortless. There are cleansing foods, building foods, and foods that cause a sugar-burning state, a protein-burning state, or a fat-burning state, and as you have learned, different foods react independently inside the body.

Step 1 outlines what foods to avoid and which to replace them with to prevent body fat and to keep the internal system clean and alkaline versus acidic.

In Step 2, you will learn what natural supplements are necessary to strengthen + maintain muscle mass from deterioration and why.

FATS:

What are fats and oils?

Fat are a collection of high-energy molecules.

Fats and oils are also known as lipids. Lipids are made up of triglycerides, which are a collection of molecules. If the lipids are liquid at room temperature, they are called oils; if they are solid at room temperature, they are called fats.

Fats are found in foods, and inside the body. Liquid or solid, fats are fats.

Saturated fatty acids are the body's natural fats. Saturated fat provides energy for the heart and muscles.

How does the body use fats?

Low-fat diets are destructive to health.

Fat supplies energy for the body, cushions the organs (muscle of the heart) and builds cell membranes. The body also uses fats to absorb vitamins.

Think of saturated fats like fuel for your body. Most diets lack the right fats. The body must be abundant with the right fats, which are saturated fats and omega-3 fatty acids. Saturated fats also keep blood sugar levels down.

The wrong fats that only cause damage to health and deplete energy levels ought to be cut out completely.

Saturated fats are found in all the human cell membranes. Saturated fats are the steadiest source of fuel for the body. They act as carriers for fat-soluble vitamins, which are pivotal for nutrient absorption and metabolism.

The proper fat consumption is a critical source of fuel for the body and for overall health.

Coconut oil:

Coconut oil is the most stable saturated fat in the fat family. Sugars and starches would be fast burning, dirty fuels that spike blood sugar levels (sugar-burning state.) If your body kicks into a sugar-burning state, muscle mass will regress. To maintain muscle mass from deterioration and to avoid excess fat accumulation, the body must use saturated fats as a source of fuel.

Coconut oil provides a steady concentrated source of fuel. The most stable, cleanest source of saturated fat in existence, coconut oil stabilizes blood sugar levels (crucial to maintaining muscle mass) because it's made of a medium chain triglyceride, or MCT. MCT is used by the body as energy without spiking the blood insulin. Coconut oil stabilize blood sugar levels, and it sustains body energy for peak performance. Coconut oil is also the slowest most sustainable source of fuel for the body (fat-burning state).

Benefits of coconut oil:

Coconut oil carries benefits beyond what most might understand.

- Reduces risk of heart disease

- Cures kidney infection and protects the liver

- Lauric acid keeps the internal system clean

- Lauric acid counters 'starvation mode'

- Fatty acids found in coconut oil kills and prevents fungal overgrowth

- Improves memory

- Improves endurance and boosts energy levels

- Improves all types of skin conditions

- Fights and prevents osteoporosis

Note: Most coconut oil on the market comes from the coconut's interior flesh known as copra, which has been heated to separate the solid interior of the coconut from the oil. Then the remaining oil goes into a further heating process to burn off any moisture and more heating to further isolate the oil. This is the coconut oil to avoid.

Coconut oil that hasn't been refined or heated or processed is the correct one to take. Unrefined, preserved of saturated fat, with high levels of MCT, cold-pressed coconut oil is the right choice to tone muscle and to burn excess body fat.

Cold-pressed means the oil has been extracted from the seed of the grain without being heated in high temperatures and solvents.

Chronic fat-burning state:

In the category of proteins, fats, and carbohydrates, carbohydrates are what the body prefers to use as fuel.

Carbohydrates are the number one source of fuel for the human body. They burn smoothly without causing acid buildup, but they burn fast and are unable to sustain muscle. Simple carbohydrates like honey, syrup, and fruit sugars burn the fastest but also cause spikes of blood sugar levels if consumed in excess.

Fiber-rich carbohydrates, like raw vegetables, burn the slowest. The more raw vegetables and green drinks (cleansing foods) that are consumed, the better the digestion and fast bowel movements.

However, raw vegetables alone are inadequate to sustain muscle mass. A highly alkaline diet is necessary for peak performance but insufficient to maintain muscle mass and for the body to use as a source of fuel. The key is to add saturated fats from coconut oil to your diet to sustain muscle mass and prevent any muscle loss. **Coconut oil is what burns the slowest, cleanest, and sustains a clean fuel source for hours at a time.**

Note: Some certified nutritionists label saturated fats as the enemy fat that causes heart disease, raises cholesterol levels and clogs the arteries. This statement couldn't be more false. Saturated fat causing heart disease was originated as a marketing propaganda to sell oils and margarine.

Coronary Heart Disease:

For over 40 years, the debate over oils, fats, and cholesterol has persisted. All doctors, nutritionist, and most health-related scholar have firmly agreed upon the following points.

1. Natural fats and oils cause heart disease.

2. Food that contains cholesterol causes heart disease.

3. Poly-unsaturated oils have the opposite effect, and would cure and prevent heart disease.

This goes to show the power of advertisement influencing people's thoughts and decisions. The rumors had spread from doctor to doctor, nutritionist to nutritionist, and eventually escalated to the media, newspapers, etc. As a result, everyone and anyone (including the media) have been brainwashed to believe that natural saturated fats and cholesterol are the foes.

Evidence:

Professor Walter Willet from Harvard:

"The focus of dietary recommendations is usually a reduction of saturated fat intake, no relation between saturated fat intake and risk of Coronary Heart Disease was observed in the most informative prospective study to date." (Willet 1990)

Doctor William P. Castelli, the director from 'Framingham Study' shares the results:

"In Framingham, for example, we found that people who ate the most cholesterol, ate the most saturated fat, ate the most calories, weighed the least, and were most physically active." (Castelli 1992)

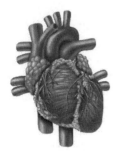

Coconut oils and fish oils are known to reduce acute and chronic inflammatory diseases. The high levels of IL-10 produced from coconut oils specially lowers inflammatory issues. IL-10 also known as Interleukin 10, is an anti-inflammatory cytokine.

More evidence from 100 years ago:

The average diet in the year 1890 was extremely high in fats. Daily meals were large, and people were more physically healthy and active. Hydrogenated oils were first brought to North America in the early 1900s. Prior to this time, there were rarely any cases of any kind of heart disease. In the decades since, heart disease has become the number one cause of early deaths and deaths in general.

One of the most preferred sources of food for the heart is saturated fat due to its steady source of fuel. Actually, the heart withdraws from the reserve of its cushioned saturated fat from muscles surrounding the heart.

The oils that cause scarring to the arteries and clog heart functions are hydrogenated, partially hydrogenated oils and omega-6 fats unbalanced with omega-3 fats. They thicken the blood, which leads to poor blood circulation, which leads to an entire army of disease and health problems.
Hydrogenation began for the sole reason to increase shelf life only.

If you are interested in learning in detail about saturated fats, unsaturated fats, cholesterol, animal fats, and digestion check out *Know Your Fats* by Mary G Enig.

Lauric acid:

Coconut oil is also known as lauric fat. Lauric acid is found in human milk for the formation for the infant. Lauric acid is one of the good fats required for the body to function. For bodybuilding and losing weight, lauric acid prevents us from going into starvation. By taking the proper doses of lauric fat, you won't feel hungry as often (which is a good thing).

Back to coconut oil:

Coconut oil is perfect for bodybuilding and weight loss because it stabilizes blood sugar levels and provides a clean sustained energy for long periods of time.

If blood sugars level remain low, you cannot gain excess body fat or lose muscle mass. Just consuming coconut oil and L-glutamine will burn off a lot of body fat. If you want to lose body fat and maintain muscle mass, coconut oil is without question a requisite in your diet.

More benefits of coconut oil related to sustaining muscle mass and burning fat:

- Prevents blood sugar levels from spiking
- Boosts levels of energy
- Enhances absorption of calcium and magnesium
- Prevents going to a sugar-burning state
- Improves digestion
- Increases metabolic rate
- Prevents further body fattening due to metabolic rate
- Keeps blood sugar levels low

Consume 6 - 7 tablespoons of coconut oil a day. Either eat the coconut oil directly or use the coconut oil as salad dressing, spread on bread, sprinkle on food, use as dip for bread or vegetables, or use frozen coconut oil as a sprinkle dressing. Be creative and use the method that works best for you.

Don't be afraid to experiment with doses of coconut oil. Think about this, the heated vegetable oils that most people consume already surpass 7-15 tablespoons or more a day. Compared to that, consuming 6+ tablespoons of coconut oil is nothing. Listen to your body and observe how your body responds to coconut oil.

Most fats found in grocery stores or supermarkets have all been refined and processed.

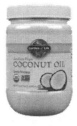

Garden of Life Organic Extra Virgin Coconut Oil, 29 oz $14.42

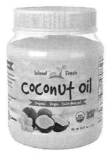

Island Fresh Superior Organic Virgin Coconut Oil, 54 Ounce $16.79

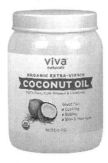

Viva Naturals Organic Extra Virgin Coconut Oil, 54 Ounce $21.75

The products I use are based on the best results I got. I will never recommend a natural supplement I haven't tested on myself. Don't believe what I say; test coconut oil out for yourself, and experience the change.

There are many studies from health experts that teach fats are unhealthy. This is true to some extent, such as the wrong fats like hydrogenated oils, partially hydrogenated oils, rancid oils, etc. Your diet must be high in saturated fats and omega 3 balanced with omega 6 oils in a 6:3 ratio which are the right fats. The key is results. If your goal is to build muscles and maintain a slim physique, saturated fats from coconut oil is the way to go.

Saturated fat and body fat accumulation:

In the category of carbohydrates, fat and protein, fats are the least fattening for the system. The reason is because fats, especially coconut oil, keep blood sugars down, unlike refined carbohydrates.

Studies have shown that coconut oil increases metabolic rate; that is to say, coconut oil enhances rapid body fat loss. Taking doses of coconut oil combined with L-glutamine burned off my body fat and increased muscle mass in a matter of weeks!

Due to coconut oil reducing blood sugar levels so intensely, sugar cravings will be reduced, if not diminished all together. Coconut oil will supply more energy for the body than caffeine, sugar, or chocolate candy ever will.

Cholesterol:

Never fear cholesterol.

Cholesterol containing foods = a healthier body. Here is why:

Cholesterol is the most misunderstood molecule of all molecules. Cholesterol is referred to as a fat. In reality,

it's a high molecule weight alcohol. The human brain in largely made of saturated fats and cholesterol. Children who consume less to little cholesterol during infancy, run the risk of suffering from cognitive brain issues. The body heals its wounds by the use of cholesterol (hint: muscle repair need cholesterol.) Human milk is loaded with high volumes of cholesterol.

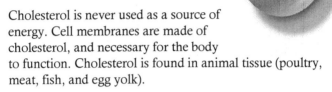

Cholesterol is never used as a source of energy. Cell membranes are made of cholesterol, and necessary for the body to function. Cholesterol is found in animal tissue (poultry, meat, fish, and egg yolk).

Note: Eggs are like the period of a chicken. We can eat eggs and still be considered a vegetarian.

When there is little cholesterol present in our diets, the body's synthesis level declines. As strict vegetarians who eat zero cholesterol, interestingly enough, the body is able to manufacture its own cholesterol called cholesterol synthesis. If cholesterol isn't provided by our diets, the liver will make cholesterol using protein, carbohydrates and fats.

What about cholesterol and heart disease?

This idea is as false as saturated fats causing heart disease. Fatty acids found in cholesterol esters are un-saturated (74% unsaturated fat).

Hydrogenated oils and omega-6 oils out of balance with omega-3 oils is what causes heart disease.

Lack of cholesterol in our diet is the most unwise choice ever.

Solution: Eat 1 or more eggs a day.

Hydrogenated oil:

Hydrogenation is the process in which chemical alteration causes unsaturated vegetable oils to have a prolonged shelf life. The vegetable oils are heated in high temperatures together with hydrogen atoms; this process creates the most toxic form of fatty acid. Hydrogenated oils are only one molecule in apart from plastic and actually closer to plastic than their natural oil counterpart. All deep-fried foods and everything oil-cooked from restaurants includes hydrogenated oils. Hydrogenated and partially hydrogenated oils must be cut out completely for the duration of the program, or cut out the harmful oils from your diet forever.

Harmful fats to avoid:

Hydrogenated fats/oils: The most toxic form of oil in existence.

Partially hydrogenated fats/oils: Causes the same harm as hydrogenated oil.

Rancid fats/oils: Processed fats that have been heated and exposed to light and oxygen and as a result turn rancid.

Processed fats: Causes the same harm as rancid fats.

Refined fats: Unnatural fats that cannot be found in nature.

Read the label of all the oils you have and purchase. Any oil that are outdated, or rancid, throw out. Any oils labeled hydrogenated, or partially hydrogenated, throw out. The same goes for refined and processed oils.

Frying with coconut oil is ok.

Replace unhealthy cooking vegetable oils with coconut oil, and healthy oils for cooking. Rotate the healthy oils over time.

To sum up fats:

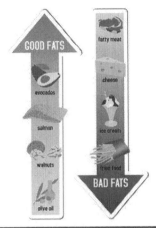

GOOD FATS vs. BAD FATS

The proper fat intake is super important for bodybuilding and health.

Fats provide a steady source of fuel for the body. They are used for mineral absorption, metabolic processes and as building blocks for cell membranes.

Low-fat diets are detrimental. Abundant quantities of the **right fats** are needed for the body to function. If you are an athlete or into bodybuilding or weight loss, your body will need even more fats.

The body requires a balance of omega 3, omega 6 and omega 9 essential fatty acids. Most diets are high in omega 6 and omega 9 fats. Types of oils high in omega 6 include olive, safflower, sunflower, soybean, sesame, borage, primrose, and canola, as well as oils made from nuts and seeds. Fats that are high in omega 3 oils include borage, hemp, flax, cod liver oil, cold water fish oils from salmon, sardines, trout and mackerel.

Cooking with some olive oil is fine.

The key is to have the fats in balance. Omega-3, omega-6 and fats are necessary. Health problems occur when fats are consumed out of balance. If only omega-3 fats are ingested over a long period of time, you will develop omega-6 deficiencies. If you ingest too much omega-6 fat, you will develop omega-3 deficiencies. The following symptoms will show up if the fat ratios become chronically out of balance.

Fats consumption ratio:

2 parts omega-3 oils, and 1 part omega-6. (6:3 ratio)

The majority of the diets people consume looks more like 1 part omega-3 to 20 parts omega-6.

Do not be concerned about taking too much coconut oil or omega 3 fats.

Most if not all diets nowadays are fully packed with omega-6 and severely lacks omega-3.

More on omega 3 - 6 - 9:

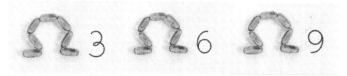

This is another area there is confusion. The balance of omega-3 and omega-6 fats is more important than most people may realize.

Why balance omega 3 – 6 with diet and supplementation?

Omega-3 fats will go a long way in maintaining muscle mass and burning body fat. Saturated fats from coconut oil and omega-3 fats work synergistically as a team. Coconut oil protects the omega-3 from oxidizing.

What does *omega* mean?

Fatty acids are separated by the families they belong to. The label omega is the specific family.

What does *essential* mean?

Oil that must be provided externally. The body cannot produce essential oils on its own.

Omega-3:

18 carbons long, has 3 double bonds, and is an essential fatty acid.

Omega-6:

18 carbons long, has 2 double bonds, and is an essential acid.

Omega-9:

Is an oleic acid. In the omega 9 family, the fatty acids are desaturated or elongated. Omega 9 fatty acids are Non-Essential, meaning the body produces omega 9 fats.

Too much omega-6 and a lack of omega-3 causes inflammation, especially heart disease.

All diseases ending in *-itis* means inflammation, which is caused by an imbalance of omega-3 fats.

- Arthritis
- Bronchitis
- Colitis
- Conjunctivitis
- Vulvitis
- Vasculitis
- Zitis
- Thyroiditis
- Keratisis
- and the list goes on...

Correct ratio 6:3:

The correct balance is 6:3 ratio. 6 of omega-3, and 3 of omega-6. Most common diets in the Western world, the ratio is 1:20+. ...1 omega-3 and 20+... omega-6.

Why is the ratio 1:20 for omega-6?

Because most people eat foods that are densely rich with omega-6 fatty acids. All foods nowadays are cooked using processed hydrogenated vegetable oils. The most common oils are soybean oil and corn oil, which are both extremely high in omega-6.

What happens then?

The shift of balance favoring omega-6 fats will cause inflammation, heart disease and strokes. 100 years ago, there were seldom if any cases of heart disease. Now, 8/10 or more of early deaths, the number one cause of early death is related to the heart.

Solution:

Eat less foods cooked by processed oils. Eat more omega-3 fatty acids. Omega-3s are found in fish, and fish oils like tuna, mackerel, and salmon. More importantly, since we are already getting so much omega-6, the best solution would be to acutely (**drastically** lower) decrease omega-6 intake, and supplement omega 3-6-9, especially omega-3 fatty acids.

Omega 3 fats:

flaxseed oil

canola oil

walnut oil

soybean oil

herring fish oil

mackerel fish oil

sardine fish oil

Omega 6 fats:

sunflower

evening primrose oil

corn oil

borage oil

olive oil

canola oil

flaxseed oil

Omega oils supplementation:

Consuming oils from and extracted source is fine, as long as the oils have been extracted properly. A number of nutritionists advise to take only omega-3 oils. In my studies, as long as we take more omega-3 vs omega-6, all is A-ok. The reason is due to the fact that the omega-6 oils most people intake are hydrogenated, rancid, damaged, etc. By supplementing with clean omega-6 fatty acids, our bodies will benefit.

Flax oil contains omega 3 – 6 – 9 in 6:3 ratio.

Directions:

Take 2 - 3 tablespoons a day.

If you're under 90 kg (200 lb) take 2 tablespoons,

If you're over 90 kg (200 lb) take 3 tablespoons.

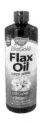

Nature's Way EFA Gold Flax Oil Super Lignan – 24 oz **$13.22**

If you feel like you have balanced omega-3 and 6 in your diet, and would like omega-3 alone, take cod liver oil. Taking cod liver oil together with flax oil is even better.

Cod liver oil only contains only omega-3.

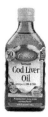

Carlson Labs Cod Liver Oil Lemon 500ml **$32.44**

Directions:

Take 2 - 3 table spoons a day.

If you're under 90 kg (200 lb) take 1-2 tablespoons,

If you're over 90 kg (200 lb) take 2-3 tablespoons.

MAGNESIUM + CALCIUM

Consuming cow milk and dairy products is counterproductive to the skeleton and overall health. Know that bone deterioration is FAR worse than muscle deterioration. The skeleton is comparative to pillars of the body. In my experience, food alone doesn't provide the proper nutrients for the bones, especially teeth. However, that does not mean magnesium and calcium supplements have been chemically manufactured. The best way to strengthen the muscles and bones is by combining calcium with magnesium.

Magnesium is rare in foods. Magnesium also controls hormone production in the body. Magnesium drastically reduces PMS symptoms most females suffer due to hormone imbalances when consumed together with calcium. Spinach is packed with magnesium. The best way to absorb magnesium is from green drinks from organic vegetables.

Magnesium and calcium work synergistically.

There are countless benefits of magnesium combined with calcium. Here are a few:

- Strengthens the bones

- Improves the texture and smoothness of the skin

- Decreases levels of stress (emotions can be destructive to health)

Calcium condenses the muscles of the body, forcing the muscles to work. Magnesium on the other hand has the opposite effect, causing the muscles to loosen up. Strengthening and toning the muscles of the body requires contraction and relaxation. Magnesium and calcium function synergistically for weight loss and to strengthen muscles.

Other benefits:

- Prevents loss of stamina

- Reduces tooth decay

- Prevents muscle cramps

- Prevents high blood pressure

- Prevents migraine headaches

- Prevents osteoporosis (weakness of bones)

- Strengthens fragile teeth

- Strengthen fragile skeleton

- Prevents muscle weakness

- Improves sleep

Most green raw vegetables carry magnesium.

There are two types of supplements to take when it comes down to magnesium.

Inorganic + ionic— **avoid.**

Organic + chelated— **take**. Best consumed by the body; it includes aspartate and orotate.

Here are two supplements that work fine:

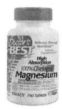

Doctor's Best High Absorption Magnesium (200 Mg Elemental), 240 Tablets **$15.38**

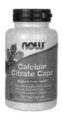

Now Foods, Calcium Citrate, 250 Tablets **$14.55**

Taking magnesium at night before bed is the best time. Magnesium soothes the muscles and makes sleep a more superior experience.

MOST ABUNDANT AMINO ACID: L-GLUTAMINE

Amino acids are the building blocks of life.

There are 20 amino acids known as the standard amino acids necessary for the human body. These amino acids can be divided into three groups: essential, semi-essential and non-essential. Some of these amino acids cannot be produced by the human body and need to be supplied externally either through foods or supplementation.

The amino acids labeled L- are the only amino acid structure natural to the body, also called proteinogen amino acids. Glutamine is a non-essential amino acid found in proteins in plant-based structures.

L-glutamine is the most abundant amino acid found in the human body.

The human body requires amino acids to

- Enhance digestion
- Improve gastrointestinal health
- Act as a band-aid, protecting the intestines from further damage
- Balance mucus production and prevents diarrhea
- Improve recovery from exercise
- Improve and keeps down blood sugar levels
- Improve metabolism
- Repair body tissue
- Repair damaged bowel lining (leaky gut)

- Reduce inflammation in intestinal lining

- Protect intestinal walls and repel irritants

- Repair and regenerate muscles after strenuous usage

- Synthesize and protect muscle tissue

- Produce glycogen and immune support

- Be a source of energy and stamina

L-glutamine has multiple benefits for digestion, bowels, muscle repair, muscle building, and fat loss. Think of L-glutamine as the absolutely necessary supplement to feed muscles and burn body fat.

Regenerative medicine:

Salamanders are creatures of fascination to science, especially in the field of regenerative medicine. If a salamander is cut in half into two separate pieces, it has the ability to re-grow ½ of its body and become two whole salamanders!

Humans cannot naturally re-grow an arm or any other body part, but we have the ability to regenerate the bowels. Leaky gut is common amongst pretty much everyone. Consuming the wrong, incompatible foods for years will damage the intestinal walls, which can be punctured by hundreds if not thousands of holes that leak food particles from the bowels into the system.

How can these holes be fixed?

You will have to cleanse and regenerate the intestines. But for now, back to weight loss.

L-glutamine is critical to repair leaky gut. After a major bowel cleanse, L-glutamine combined with aloe repairs the intestinal holes called leaky gut. L-glutamine repairs leaky gut holes, and it coats the intestinal cell walls acting as a repellant to allergic foods. To do so requires extensive bowel cleansing and regenerating protocols…but for now, back to fat loss.

The same principles apply to the muscles after a strenuous workout. L-glutamine **repairs/regenerates** the muscle fibers just like the intestinal walls. **Without the proper doses of L-glutamine, strengthening/toning muscles and burning body fat will be impossible.**

A few of my favorite L-glutamine supplements that deliver the best results are:

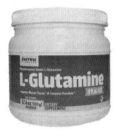

Jarrow Formulas L-Glutamine, 17.6 Oz $21.99

Directions for green drinks:

1 teaspoon of green powder + a tablespoon of fiber + inulin stevia or flavored stevia + 1 teaspoon of L-glutamine in a glass of water 3 times a day.

Note: A small percentage of people suffer from symptoms of insomnia after taking L-glutamine.

However, this is rare, and it is highly unlikely that you will suffer any kind of negative symptoms. But if your body responds negatively by taking L-glutamine, switch to amino acids from white fish instead.

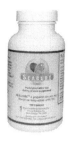

Seacure 180 Capsules $35.73

FIBER INTAKE TO SPEED UP BOWEL MOVEMENT
From the National Fiber Council:

Food	Serving Size	Grams of Fiber
Fruits		
Apple with peel-	1 medium	3
Banana-	1 medium	3
Blueberries-	1 cup	4
Cantaloupe-	1 cup	1
Grapefruit-	1 medium	1
Orange-	1 medium	3
Pear with peel-	1 medium	4
Vegetables and Beans		
Asparagus, 5 medium cooked-	½ cup	2
Kidney beans cooked-	½ cup	6
Pinto beans-	½ cup	8
Broccoli cooked-	½ cup	2
Carrots-	½ cup	2

The average amount of fiber consumed by most people is 10 grams or less a day. Fiber intake should be three to four times more than what the average person consumes. Counting grams can be extremely confusing, and it makes working out an undesirable chore. Instead, listen to your body. Two to three bowel movements a day should be enough to keep the system clean and free of waste.

To increase doses of fiber, ingest foods with high fiber content like non-starchy, raw, green leafy vegetables and fruits and keep starches, refined foods and high-protein foods low. Eating large quantities of raw vegetables should provide most of the fiber needed. In addition, by adding fiber from fiber supplements, bowel transit time will increase many times over.

Mucoid plaque buildup in the bowels will slow down bowel transit time regardless of how much fiber is consumed. That is why it is crucial to perform a deep internal detoxification for optimal health. Backed up bowels will pollute the system like nothing else.

Proper doses of fiber are crucial to remove old waste quickly from the bowels. In addition, proper doses of fiber slow down the pace of sugar entering the blood stream, keeping blood sugar levels low. Fiber can be found in seeds, fruits, leaves, and stems.

Even the purest raw vegetables will rot if they sit in the bowels for long periods of time. Fiber is like a vacuum cleaner, absorbing all toxins and cleaning up outdated digested foods in the GI tract's path.

Fiber is the solution to speed up bowel movements and to destroy toxin buildup in the colon.

Factors that determine rapid bowel movements:

- Amount of fiber consumed.

- Lack or amount of mucoid plaque buildup in the bowels.

- Consumption or lack of consumption of protein powder, high concentration protein foods and system-clogging foods.

The body building community often recommends protein powder, but it is extremely acid-forming in the system, it hinders digestion and it slows down bowel transit time.

Whey protein and casein protein shakes do nothing but clog, harm and cause disease.

Raw vegetables + green drinks are packed with fibers.

Refined grains + refined carbohydrates have zero fiber.

To speed up bowel transit time, simply add some psyllium husk fiber into your green drink or water.

The best soluble fiber supplements to eliminate waste fast and to keep the colon clean is psyllium husk:

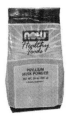

Now Foods Psyllium Husk Powder, 24 oz $15.29

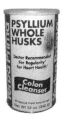

Yerba Prima, Psyllium Whole Husks, Colon Cleanser, 12 oz (340 g) $11.36

Here are two of my favorite fiber supplements that I use to keep my bowels clean and free of waste.

Make sure to look for "soluble fiber" as opposed to "insoluble fiber." Just as it sounds, soluble fiber dissolves in water, and insoluble does not. Soluble fiber is most effective in cleaning out the colons of toxins. Insoluble fiber doesn't do the job as effectively.

Soluble fiber also feeds on friendly bacteria to make it grow + multiply.

STEP 3. HOW TO FIRE UP DIGESTION

Digestion explained:

If digestion is strong, fast and easy, then strengthening the muscles and burning fat will be strong, fast and easy.

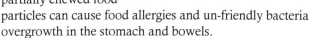

How food is consumed is more important than which foods are eaten. If food isn't properly chewed or if you drink liquid together with solid foods, the body will have trouble digesting. Un-chewed or partially chewed food particles can cause food allergies and un-friendly bacteria overgrowth in the stomach and bowels.

Digestion → absorption → elimination

Mouth: Digestive juices in the saliva mixed with food travels to the stomach where food is broken down.

Stomach: Where digestion occurs.

Small intestines: Responsible for absorption.

Colon: Excretes leftovers as waste.

The goal is to digest fast, digest properly, digest completely, and have old waste removed quickly for a new digestion session to begin.

As you have learned, eating 4-6 small meals a day will not only force the body into a sugar-burning state, but it will majorly interrupt digestion. Allow digestion to finish before eating another meal session.

Note: Overly stuffing yourself with food at one time will hinder digestion. Listen to your body, eat enough food until you're full, but avoid over-eating.

Drink fluids at times when you are not eating food

If you drink fluids together with solid foods, the digestive fluids responsible for breaking down food particles will be severely compromised. This will put a heavy burden on digestion, and slow down digestion by many folds.

Water and fluids are necessary for the body to stay hydrated and for detoxification. Drink fluids separately, at least half an hour apart from meals. Supplements must be consumed one hour apart. Green drinks and supplementation should be consumed in between, before or after meals.

If you are eating spicy foods or dry foods, or if you require water for any other reason, a sip of water before or after a meal is all that's necessary.

Chew food completely

This is the simplest yet most crucial part of digestion. In order for the digestive fluids to break down food, the food must be chewed into its tiniest pieces. The slower and more completely food is chewed, the faster digestion will flow. Large, undigested food chunks will upset the stomach and cause acid buildup, and putrefy like nothing else.

Break down/chew the food inside the mouth extremely slowly, into the smallest pieces possible before swallowing. Take time to complete each meal.

Fully digest before exercise

If someone exercises shortly after a large meal, the body will be kicked out of digesting mode and go into active mode. In other words, blood required to digest moves towards the muscles.

After a meal, the body requires time to digest completely before any kind of heavy lifting or exercise.

Wait a couple of hours for digestion to complete before doing any kind of strenuous exercise.

Remember the analogy of the dishwasher? Fully allow digestion to complete before eating any more food or strenuous movement. By eating 2-3 large meals a day combined with coconut oil, your body will burn fats as fuel and digestion will remain strong.

Cycles of the body and nature

Everything in nature functions in cycles.

Winter → spring → summer → fall and the cycle repeats over and over again.

Life cycles, harvesting cycles, monthly cycles, daily cycles...everything in this world functions in cycles, including the human body, which goes through a cleansing, assimilation and absorption cycle every day.

For the body to cleanse, digest or assimilate, these cycles require a lot of energy. You must learn to work together with your body's natural cycles as opposed to going against them.

Cleansing cycle:

Cleansing cycle: 5:00 am to 10:00 am (early morning) is when the body expels toxins from the system. Taking supplements, green drinks and some fruits or snacks is fine during this time. However, avoid eating the bulk of the day's meals.

Absorption cycle: 10:00 am to 7:00 pm (mid-afternoon) is when the body requires nutrients or absorption time. This is the ideal time when nature has designed the body to consume food and nutrients. Two to three large meals have to be consumed during the absorption cycle.

Assimilation cycle: 7:00 pm–11 pm (evening) is the time when the body assimilates nutrients, providing energy to separate organs and cells. It is fine to consume supplements during this time, but stay away from heavy meals.

If you form a habit of eating meals during the cleansing cycle or assimilation cycle, the body can lead to chronic toxic build up and cause malfunction in the long run. Allow your body to cleanse and assimilate as it was designed.

How to fire up digestion x2

This simple yet powerful method allows the stomach to digest food more completely, and speeds up the digestion process x2.

The method is highly effective. And the answer is to eat a fresh slice of ginger before or after a meal with a sip of water.

Ginger can be found in most grocery stores. Eating a small piece before or after a meal together with some water will stimulate digestion x2.

Note: I did not say drink cups of water together with ginger after a meal.

For a test, stand in front of a mirror and stick out your tongue. If your tongue has a white coating, this is an indication of 3 things:

1. Week digestion.
2. Mucoid plaque buildup.
3. Fungal and mold overgrowth.

As you consume a slice of ginger before or after a large meal, keep an eye on your tongue. In a few days, the tongue will change into a healthy red color.

Remember, to strengthen muscle tone, digestion must be complete and strong.

Step 4: TRANSPLANT FRIENDLY BACTERIA

Absorption of nutrients occurs in the small and large intestinal walls. Friendly bacteria maintain the colon at proper pH levels, prevent fungal growth, and help the assimilation of nutrition.

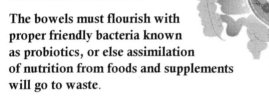

The bowels must flourish with proper friendly bacteria known as probiotics, or else assimilation of nutrition from foods and supplements will go to waste.

How are friendly bacteria transplanted into the bowels?

- Bowels cannot be acidic
- Bowels must be alkaline
- Cannot be on antibiotics (worst enemy of probiotics that will wipe out friendly intestinal flora entirely)

Note: The best way to transplant probiotics is during/after a deep internal detoxification cleanse.

If you're following the diet as outlined in the "what to eat" section, your bowels should be free of acidity and they should be alkaline and ready to transplant intestinal flora.

However, this isn't the entire battle. Think of transplanting friendly bacteria as a war. Currently, unfriendly bacteria have colonized the land (stomach, small intestines, large intestines), which must be re-colonized by friendly bacteria. For the friendly army to successfully colonize the bowels, a large and powerful army must be sent to the battle front to completely wipeout and replace the non-friendly bacteria army.

Most probiotic supplements made of acidophilus will die off shortly after consumption inside the stomach before it can reach the intestines. Probiotics are very fragile, and most probiotic supplements do not implant at all or die fairly rapidly.

Lactobifudus and streptococcus are what implant for long periods of time and most effortlessly.

Here's the best probiotic that contains lactobifudus and streptococcus, stay alive and flourish inside the bowels for months at a time.

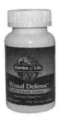

Garden of Life, Primal Defense, HSO Probiotic Formula, 90 Veggie Caplets $26.49

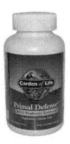

Garden of Life, Primal Defense, HSO Probiotic Formula, 216 Caplets $51.90

Consume 6 or more caplets with lots of water + fiber in the morning or evening on an empty stomach for at least 3 weeks or longer. Don't be afraid to experiment. Remember, think of colonizing friendly bacteria as an army would invade enemy grounds.

To keep your bowels fully colonized, have a transplant session every 6 months.

Inulin (FOS)

As you have learned, probiotics are very fragile, and they need their own source of food to flourish. Fiber feeds on friendly bacteria. There is a special fiber by the name of fructooligosaccharides (FOS), also known as inulin, that causes insane overgrowth of the intestinal flora.

Add some inulin stevia to your drinks or foods. Here are two of my favorite inulin stevia products that come in powder form. Again, experiment with the stevia doses and products.

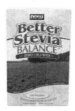

Now Foods, Better Stevia Balance, Zero Calories, 100 Packets, (1.1 g) Each $10.35

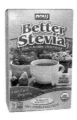

Now Foods, Organic, Better Stevia, Zero Calorie Sweetener, 75 Packets, 2.65 oz (75 g) $5.60

To wrap and finish up

IF YOU FOLLOW THESE PRINCIPLES, YOU ARE
GURANTEED TO BURN BODY FAT COMPLETELY
AND MAINTAIN A SLIM PHYSIQUE PERMANENTLY.

The information in this text is most likely new. You must
have an open mind, be open to new ideas, and let go of
incorrect programming and old habits to achieve any measure
of success in weight loss and in your life. If you continue to
conform and follow the follower, you will never be able to
achieve any new results.

Before we move onto the workout…

There is only one person in this entire planet everybody
thinks, cares, talks about 99.99999% of the time.

Do you know who that person is? You!

Everyone only cares about themselves.

This makes sense, because everyone is responsible for
themselves, and if each individual doesn't take care of
themselves…who would?

However, people who are only self-centered or self-motivated
may achieve all if not most of their *external goals* and may feel
an uplift in their mood, happiness and success, but it is only
temporary.

People who are happiest and driven by *internal goals* sustain
their motivation and happiness for long periods of time.

What are internal goals?

If you really understand that every person in this world is on
the same boat, on the same earth separated in individual
bodies, and if you come to realize that we are dependent on
each other for our well-being and survival, real rewards don't
come from accumulation or acquiring, but by giving.

Adding more value, meeting the needs of other people, and solving their issues/struggles/problems will lead to infinite fulfillment, happiness and permanent success.

If you know a friend who struggles to lose weight or build muscle, share this program with him or her. And know and feel that making a difference in other people's lives is far more rewarding than making a difference in your own.

BONUS #2:

Workout Routine:

Note: If you don't have access to a gym for whatever reason or are a complete beginner, start by working out at home with bodyweight exercises. By signing up for the Bonus #3 newsletter, I will give you the best bodyweight home workout for FREE.

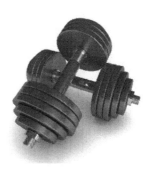

Caution: If you have little experience lifting weights, you must begin by learning how to lift weights from a physical trainer. Beginners are at high risk of injury if you do not know how to pump iron.

Ask the physical trainer at your local gym to spot you a couple of times and to give you some basic workout advice. The fitness instructors at your gym will not have the information you have now. If they give you tips on nutrition and what to eat, suggesting protein shakes, -6 small meals a day, etc., pretend to listen to them, chuckle, and move onto your workout.

Don't argue or try to straighten out their thinking. Let them do whatever they desire to, because soon they will be asking you for nutrition and workout advice!

But seriously, in the beginning, you must learn how to pump iron first from a fitness instructor or from an experienced friend.

Back to business...

Burning body fat is simple. You have to understand the difference between building muscle mass for bodybuilders and lifting weights to tone/strengthen muscles in order to burn excess body fat.

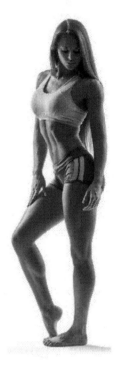

Bodybuilders lift less reps and steadily increase weights. They increase the weights and pump until failure (until the body cannot lift/handle anymore). Only by forcefully tearing and ripping the muscles, muscle mass will increase in size.

To burn body fat, you must lift light weights, steadily increase the weights over time, but don't lift until failure and do more reps. Your attitude should be, "I feel a satisfactory pump after the 20 reps." Pump until you feel like you are done.

To burn fat:

20-22 reps, 3 sets.

You must listen to your body. Use this workout routine by how you feel, by how your body responds.

How to lift weights:

In the beginning, you must try out each of the workouts to know the exact weights to lift per session. Carry a notepad and pen with you to the gym, and write down which exercise + weights + sets and reps, and the date. The next workout session, you will know how much you lifted in the previous session, and steadily increase or decrease weights (if necessary) from there until you can achieve 3 sets of 20 reps per workout.

The answer is to be able to do 3 sets of 20 reps.

Example:

- If you are going to lift 5kg (11 pounds) barbell bench press— 2.5kg (5.5 pounds) on each side of the barbell, and can only manage 15 reps → **then lower the weights to a total of 4kg** (8.8 pounds) **or 3kg** (6.6 pounds), and attempt again until 20 reps are manageable per set.

- You must listen to your body.

- Gradually increase the weights as the weeks go on.

- Before a set, program yourself to do 22 reps (intensity of the pump) when aiming for a total of 20.

- If the current weights you are lifting feel too light, increase the weights until you are able to manage a total of 3 sets of 20 reps.

  o You have to listen to your body. Lifting 3 sets of 20 reps for each exercise is sufficient.

  o The intensity of the pump is what strengthens/tones muscles.

  o Only 20-40 minutes or less should be spent at the gym per workout session.

The same mistakes made by bodybuilders also apply to weight loss:

Chronic repetition of the same workout.

- Lifting weights forces the muscles to use fibers that wouldn't normally be used.

- If the same muscle fibers are repetitively worked out without alternation, the body will become accustomed to, or become immune to the same workout.

- Exercises must be alternated during each workout session when hitting the same body part.

Example:

Chest workout

1st workout session:
- Barbell bench press wide grip
- Dumbbell fly

2nd workout session:
- Incline dumbbell press
- Flat bench cable fly

3rd workout session:
- Dumbbell press
- Dumbbell fly

4th workout session:
- Barbell incline bench press
- Flat bench cable fly

5th workout session: *Return to 1st workout, and continue the cycle.*

Here I have created a two-week workout program, pumping six days a week and resting only once. This may seem like working out too often, but know that you're only spending 40-20 minutes **or less** at the gym per session.

Use this workout schedule as a guide, and design your own workout routine according to **how your body responds**. If working out six days a week is too strenuous, start by pumping three days a week. Again, you must listen to your body.

If your shoulders are sore when it's shoulder/back/lats day, do some cardio or abs or workout a distinct body part or rest all together. You must listen to your body; I cannot emphasize this enough. Make your body a friend, not an enemy.

1st week:

Mon
(chest/triceps/bicep)
1. Barbell bench-press
2. Dumbbell fly
3. Lying close-up barbell triceps
4. Alternate incline dumbbell curl

Tue
(legs/glutes)
1. Barbell full squat
2. Flutter kick

Wed
(shoulder/back/lats)
1. Dumbbell shoulder
2. Bent-over two arm long bar row
3. Wide grip rear pull up

Thur
REST

Fri
(chest/triceps/bicep)
1. Incline dumbbell press
2. Flat bench cable fly
3. Tricep dumbbell kickback
4. 4. EZ-bar curl

Sat
(leg)
1. Leg extension
2. Lying leg curl
3. Seated calf raise

Sun
(shoulder/back/lats)
1. Seated bent over over rear delt raise
2. Front dumbell raise
3. Seated cable rows
4. Wide grip rear pull up

2nd week:

Mon
(chest/triceps/bicep)
1. Dumbbell bench press
2. Dumbbell fly
3. Kneeling tricep cable extension
4. Alternate incline dumbbell curl

Tue
(legs/glutes)
1. Leg extension
2. Lying leg curl
3. Flutter kick
4. Seated calf raise

Wed
(shoulder/back/lats)
1. Seated side lateral raise
2. One arm dumbbell row
3. wide grip rear pull up

Thur	Fri	Sat	Sun
REST	(chest/triceps/bicep)	(leg)	(shoulder/back/lats)
	1. Incline barbell bench press	1. Barbell full squat	1. Dumbbell shoulder press
	2. Flat bench cable flyes	2. Flutter kick	2. Bent-over two arm...
	3. Lying barbell triceps extension behind the head		3. Wide grip rear pull
	4. EZ-bar curl		

Watch the video gym workout tutorials in:

www.nekoterran.com/workout

List of exercises with video tutorial on bodybuilding.com

http://www.bodybuilding.com/exercises/finder

Chest:

Barbell bench-press wide grip

Barbell incline bench-press

Dumbbell bench press

Dumbbell fly

Flat bench cable fly

Tricep:

Lying close-up barbell tricep extension behind the head

Tricep dumbbell kickback

Kneeling tricep cable extension

Bicep:

Alternate incline dumbbell curl

EZ-bar curl

Shoulder:

Dumbbell shoulder press

Seated Bent-over rear delt raise

Front dumbbell raise

Seated side lateral raise

Back:

Seated cable rows

Bent-over two arm long bar row

One arm dumbbell row

Wide-grip rear pull-up

Leg:

Barbell full squat

Flutter kick

Leg extension

Lying leg curl

Seated calf raise

Build muscle like bodybuilders:

Losing weight is easy.

Building large muscles for bodybuilders is hard.

Building big muscles without pumping iron is unattainable.

Some followers have reported having lost a considerable amount of weight without even exercising.

After completing the 8- 10 week program, chances are you will have lost 90% or more of your body fat. This can depend on several factors, such as how strict you were on the diet, if you exercised regularly, and if you pumped iron at a gym or home, etc.

To build muscle mass, keep the diet and supplements the same. At the gym, instead of doing 3 sets of 22 reps, now you will do 3 sets of 12 reps until failure.

Building big muscles requires forcefully tearing and ripping the muscles using heavier weights. To burn body fat, you are lifting lighter weights, heavy enough to complete 22 reps until satisfaction. Building muscle mass can be extremely exhausting.

Why build muscle mass?

After melting away all of your body fat, certainly some body parts will be weaker/skinnier, and out of proportion compared to the rest of the body.

For example, if your legs are too skinny, add muscle mass to your thighs and calves. Monitor your progress in the mirror.

Cardio:

By now, you might be thinking, "Isn't there any jogging in this program?"

Through my experience, the doses of L-glutamine combined with coconut oil burnt off a big portion of my body fat and bulked muscle mass even without much effort.

Digestion + diet + amino acids + coconut oil + workout will burn off 95% or more of total body fat. You can choose to do some cardio or abs after a workout session or on a rest day.

However, don't overdo it. Only 5 minutes of jogging is required until you break a sweat, then walk for 10–15 minutes. Jogging for long periods of time can deteriorate muscle mass. Just look at marathon runners vs 100-dash runners.

How to maintain muscle long-term:

As you have learned, your body requires fuel to function. If you want to maintain muscle mass and avoid deterioration, your body must always be in a fat-burning state and avoid going to a protein- or sugar-burning state.

Keep an alkaline system and green drinks a long-lasting part of your life. Only good things will come from keeping your system clean.

After the intense 8 – 10 week program, hitting each body part once a week or once every 2 weeks is sufficient to maintain muscle mass and fat accumulation.

After the 8- 10 weeks, experiment with the reps and sets or exercises and design your own workout routine.

Now you have a complete understanding of how to burn body fat completely and maintain a slim physique permanently.

Conclusion:

I have done my best for you to achieve the physique you desire to attain. For years, I struggled at the gym, leading to frustration after frustration, dead end after dead end, and wasting years of my life as I was unable to achieve any measure of success. How I wish I could have had this information when I first started out! However, if you only take in this information, absolutely nothing will happen. You must put this information into action.

The whole reason I created this program was so my readers could achieve some measure of success and happiness with their lives. It takes a lot of courage to invest and follow through with this program. Because you are reading this now, it proves to me and to yourself how powerful and determined for change you really are.

I am only successful when you (my readers) are successful.

And now the time has come to enjoy long-lasting results.

Final Note: My other program, "Intestinal Cleanse and Reconstruction," is a powerful deep internal detoxification program. Anyone over the age of 15 can be carrying 10kg (**22 pounds**) –20kg (**44 pounds**) of mucoid plaque inside their bowels that clogs and pollutes the system. You will be more successful transplanting friendly bacteria once the intestines have been cleaned out. Digestion, bowel movements, losing weight, and building muscle will be more effective once the primary channels of elimination work up to par.

Thank you for reading, and have fun building some serious muscle!

As an author, I value your reviews. It helps others to make an informed decision before reading the book. If you feel like you have gained enlightened knowledge, please consider leaving a short review in the following link.

It'd be greatly appreciated!

www.nekoterran.com/advice

Thank you and good luck!

BONUS #2: *(Absolutely a must to achieve top shape)* Sign up to receive the BEST home bodyweight workout and more health advice from me.

www.nekoterran.com/advice

All Titles B&W and Color

available at CreateSpace Store...

To learn more go to

www.Nekoterran.com

More Health & Fitness Titles:

Basic Bodybuilding

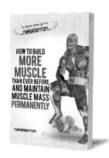

✓ What builds muscles.

✓ What causes muscle mass deterioration.

✓ What causes body fat.

✓ How to burn body fat.

✓ How to maintain muscle mass.

✓ How to maintain a fat-less physique.

✓ *Choose only basic bodybuilding or basic weight loss.*

Basic Weight Loss

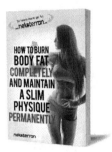

✓ What tones/strengthens muscles.

✓ What causes muscle mass deterioration.

✓ What causes body fat.

✓ How to prevent body fat.

✓ How to burn existing body fat.

✓ How to maintain muscle mass.

✓ How to maintain a fat-less physique.

✓ *Choose only basic bodybuilding or basic weight loss.*

Choose only **one** program – Weight Loss or Bodybuilding

Basic Internal Detox

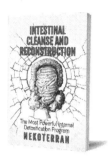

✓ Deep internal detoxification program.

✓ This is the ideal program to begin with.

✓ Complete this program first before attempting weight loss or bodybuilding basics

✓ *Works in conjunction with every other program.*

Advanced Bodybuilding

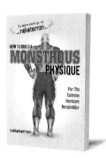

✓ For the advanced bodybuilder.

✓ The final step out of 3.

✓ *Must first complete the internal detox program.*

✓ *Must first complete the basic bodybuilding program.*

82725735R00062

Made in the USA
Middletown, DE
05 August 2018